The Personal Protective Technology Program at NIOSH

Reviews of Research Programs of the
National Institute for Occupational Safety and Health

Committee to Review the NIOSH Personal
Protective Technology Program

Board on Health Sciences Policy

INSTITUTE OF MEDICINE AND
NATIONAL RESEARCH COUNCIL
OF THE NATIONAL ACADEMIES

THE NATIONAL ACADEMIES PRESS
Washington, D.C.
www.nap.edu

THE NATIONAL ACADEMIES PRESS • 500 Fifth Street, NW • Washington, DC 20001

NOTICE: The project that is the subject of this report was approved by the Governing Board of the National Research Council, whose members are drawn from the councils of the National Academy of Sciences, the National Academy of Engineering, and the Institute of Medicine. The members of the committee responsible for the report were chosen for their special competences and with regard for appropriate balance.

This study was requested by the National Institute for Occupational Safety and Health of the Centers for Disease Control and Prevention and supported by Award No. 211-2006-19152, T.O. #1, between the National Academy of Sciences and the Centers for Disease Control and Prevention. Any opinions, findings, conclusions, or recommendations expressed in this publication are those of the author(s) and do not necessarily reflect the view of the organizations or agencies that provided support for this project.

International Standard Book Number 13: 978-0-309-12018-0
International Standard Book Number 10: 0-309-12018-7

Additional copies of this report are available from the National Academies Press, 500 Fifth Street, N.W., Lockbox 285, Washington, DC 20055; (800) 624-6242 or (202) 334-3313 (in the Washington metropolitan area); Internet, http://www.nap.edu.

For more information about the Institute of Medicine, visit the IOM home page at: **www.iom.edu**.

Copyright 2008 by the National Academy of Sciences. All rights reserved.

Printed in the United States of America

Cover credits: Photographs are reprinted with permission courtesy of DuPont and of MSA (Mine Safety Appliances Company).

Suggested Citation: Institute of Medicine and National Research Council. 2008. *The Personal Protective Technology Program at NIOSH*. Committee to Review the NIOSH Personal Protective Technology Program. Rpt. No. 5, Reviews of Research Programs of the National Institute for Occupational Safety and Health. Washington, DC: The National Academies Press.

THE NATIONAL ACADEMIES
Advisers to the Nation on Science, Engineering, and Medicine

The **National Academy of Sciences** is a private, nonprofit, self-perpetuating society of distinguished scholars engaged in scientific and engineering research, dedicated to the furtherance of science and technology and to their use for the general welfare. Upon the authority of the charter granted to it by the Congress in 1863, the Academy has a mandate that requires it to advise the federal government on scientific and technical matters. Dr. Ralph J. Cicerone is president of the National Academy of Sciences.

The **National Academy of Engineering** was established in 1964, under the charter of the National Academy of Sciences, as a parallel organization of outstanding engineers. It is autonomous in its administration and in the selection of its members, sharing with the National Academy of Sciences the responsibility for advising the federal government. The National Academy of Engineering also sponsors engineering programs aimed at meeting national needs, encourages education and research, and recognizes the superior achievements of engineers. Dr. Charles M. Vest is president of the National Academy of Engineering.

The **Institute of Medicine** was established in 1970 by the National Academy of Sciences to secure the services of eminent members of appropriate professions in the examination of policy matters pertaining to the health of the public. The Institute acts under the responsibility given to the National Academy of Sciences by its congressional charter to be an adviser to the federal government and, upon its own initiative, to identify issues of medical care, research, and education. Dr. Harvey V. Fineberg is president of the Institute of Medicine.

The **National Research Council** was organized by the National Academy of Sciences in 1916 to associate the broad community of science and technology with the Academy's purposes of furthering knowledge and advising the federal government. Functioning in accordance with general policies determined by the Academy, the Council has become the principal operating agency of both the National Academy of Sciences and the National Academy of Engineering in providing services to the government, the public, and the scientific and engineering communities. The Council is administered jointly by both Academies and the Institute of Medicine. Dr. Ralph J. Cicerone and Dr. Charles M. Vest are chair and vice chair, respectively, of the National Research Council.

www.national-academies.org

COMMITTEE TO REVIEW THE NIOSH PERSONAL PROTECTIVE TECHNOLOGY PROGRAM

E. JOHN GALLAGHER (*Chair*), University Chair, Department of Emergency Medicine, Albert Einstein College of Medicine, New York City
ROGER L. BARKER, Professor, Department of Textile Engineering, Chemistry and Science, North Carolina State University, Raleigh
HOWARD J. COHEN, Professor of Occupational Safety and Health Management, University of New Haven, CT
JANICE COMER-BRADLEY, Technical Director, International Safety Equipment Association, Arlington, VA
ELIZABETH A. CORLEY, Assistant Professor, School of Public Affairs, Arizona State University, Phoenix
RICHARD M. DUFFY, Assistant to the General President, International Association of Fire Fighters, Washington, DC
JAMES S. JOHNSON, Consultant, JSJ and Associates, Pleasanton, CA
JAMES M. MCCULLOUGH,[1] Senior Researcher, SRI International, Arlington, VA
JIMMY PERKINS, Professor, Environmental and Occupational Health, University of Texas School of Public Health, San Antonio
DAVID PREZANT, Chief Medical Officer, Office of Medical Affairs, New York City Fire Department; Professor of Medicine, Albert Einstein College of Medicine, New York City
KNUT RINGEN, Independent Consultant, Seattle, WA
EMANUEL P. RIVERS, Director of Research, Emergency Department, Henry Ford Hospital, Detroit, MI
JOSEPH J. SCHWERHA, Professor and Director of the Occupational and Environmental Medicine Residency and the Disaster Preparedness Certificate Program, University of Pittsburgh, PA
ANUGRAH SHAW, Professor, Department of Human Ecology, University of Maryland Eastern Shore, Princess Anne
TONYA SMITH-JACKSON, Associate Professor of Human Factors Engineering, Department of Industrial and Systems Engineering, Virginia Polytechnic Institute and State University, Blacksburg

Framework Committee Liaison

SUSAN E. COZZENS, Director, Technology Policy and Assessment Center, Georgia Institute of Technology, Atlanta

---

[1] Resigned from committee effective November 12, 2007.

Board on Health Sciences Policy Liaison

MARTHA HILL, Dean and Professor of Nursing, Johns Hopkins University, Baltimore, MD

Project Staff

CATHY LIVERMAN, Study Director
TOM PLEWES, Senior Program Officer
ERICKA MCGOWAN, Associate Program Officer
JUDY ESTEP, Program Associate

Independent Report Reviewers

This report has been reviewed in draft form by individuals chosen for their diverse perspectives and technical expertise, in accordance with procedures approved by the National Research Council's Report Review Committee. The purpose of this independent review is to provide candid and critical comments that will assist the institution in making its published report as sound as possible and to ensure that the report meets institutional standards for objectivity, evidence, and responsiveness to the study charge. The review comments and draft manuscript remain confidential to protect the integrity of the deliberative process. We wish to thank the following individuals for their review of this report:

Jacqueline Agnew, Department of Environmental Health Sciences, Johns Hopkins Bloomberg School of Public Health
Don B. Chaffin, Industrial and Operations Engineering and Biomedical Engineering, University of Michigan
Sarah Felknor, Southwest Center for Occupational and Environmental Health, University of Texas School of Public Health
Robert A. Freese, Globe Manufacturing Company
Zane Frund, Chemical Research and Analytical Services, Mine Safety Appliances Company
Stephan Graham, Industrial Hygiene Field Services Program, Directorate of Occupational Health Sciences, U.S. Army Center for Health Promotion and Preventive Medicine

Sundaresan Jayaraman, School of Polymer, Textile and Fiber Engineering and College of Management, Georgia Institute of Technology
Jeffery Kravitz, Scientific Development, Mine Safety and Health Administration
Fred A. Mettler, Radiology and Nuclear Medicine, New Mexico Veterans Health Care System
James W. Platner, CPWR: The Center for Construction Research and Training
Lewis J. Radonovich, Project BREATHE, and Biosecurity Programs, Office of Program Development, North Florida/South Georgia Veterans Health System
Kenneth D. Rosenman, Division of Occupational and Environmental Medicine, Michigan State University
John A. Schaefer, Health, Safety and Environment Department, Johns Hopkins University School of Medicine
Bruce Tatarchuk, Center for Microfibrous Materials Manufacturing, Department of Chemical Engineering, Auburn University

Although the reviewers listed above have provided many constructive comments and suggestions, they were not asked to endorse the conclusions or recommendations, nor did they see the final draft of the report before its release. The review of this report was overseen by **Paul D. Stolley,** University of Maryland School of Medicine, and **Kristine M. Gebbie,** Columbia University School of Nursing. Appointed by the National Research Council and Institute of Medicine, they were responsible for making certain that an independent examination of this report was carried out in accordance with institutional procedures and that all review comments were carefully considered. Responsibility for the final content of this report rests entirely with the authoring committee and the institution.

Preface

A firefighter wearing turn-out gear to avoid burn injury and using a self-contained breathing apparatus to prevent inhalation of smoke and other toxic atmospheres; an emergency responder in an encapsulated suit to protect against chemical, biological, and nuclear threats; or a healthcare provider wearing gloves, gown, and a respirator to reduce transmission of infectious diseases—these examples are prototypic of the millions of workers in a wide array of occupations who depend on personal protective technologies (PPT) for their health and safety every day.

This report provides a critical appraisal of selected features of the Personal Protective Technology Program of the National Institute for Occupational Safety and Health (NIOSH). The committee was asked to evaluate the relevance and impact of a dozen specific elements of the PPT Program in preventing work-related injury and illness, identify important future considerations for scientific investigation, and provide recommendations for program improvement. Consistent with the committee's charge from NIOSH, we focused on eight components of respiratory protection, three components of dermal protection, and a single component of injury prevention. Where relevant, we evaluated these efforts across the three domains of research, certification, and standards setting.

In conducting this study, the committee noted the significant progress that has been made in developing and testing respirators to reduce or prevent hazardous inhalation exposures, currently limited mainly by the problems of facial fit and user adherence. Concurrently the committee identified important challenges ahead in ensuring that other types of non-respiratory PPT (e.g., protective clothing, gloves, eyewear, hearing protection, helmets, and fall harnesses) receive similar attention in their testing and development. Furthermore, there are many substantive scientific and regulatory challenges in providing workers with integrated PPT that offers multiple types of necessary protection. These challenges arise because few PPT products are designed to work together in a seamless and coordinated fashion, thus causing gaps in protection where different components interface, compromising worker health and safety. In addition, PPT may be uncomfortable and may impede communication or the ability to perform one's job. Thus, as explored in detail in the report, there are a wealth of opportunities for improving PPT to better protect U.S. workers.

The impetus for a national focus on PPT gained momentum with a congressional mandate from which the National Personal Protective Technology Laboratory was created in 2001. However, the mandate was not accompanied by sufficient resources to fully implement a PPT program that could lead efforts to meet the many and varied PPT needs across all relevant occupations. The committee examined the progress the PPT Program has made in the face of limited resources, and urges implementation of our recommendations to move the entirety of this critically important area of endeavor forward.

It was a privilege to chair this committee. Truly an interdisciplinary group, its strength was in the extensive expertise, thoughtful intelligence, dedicated efforts, and unfailing good nature of its members. The committee worked diligently to provide a fair scoring of the PPT Program's relevance and impact upon worker safety and health. But rating scales have inherent limitations and it is in going beyond the scores to the narrative component of this report, particularly the five recommendations, where the committee hopes it can make a contribution to the already substantial efforts of the PPT Program.

The committee greatly benefited from the thorough briefings and informative discussions with staff members of the NIOSH PPT Program. On behalf of the committee, I want to thank Les Boord, Maryann D'Alessandro, Roland Berry Ann, Ron Shaffer, Heinz Ahlers, Jon Szalajda, Bill Haskell, Ray Sinclair, and the many other NIOSH staff who provided a wealth of information to the committee and were exceedingly patient with our sometimes insistent queries and frequent requests for clarification.

I would also like to acknowledge the extraordinary contributions made to this report by the IOM and NRC staff, specifically Cathy Liverman, Tom Plewes, Ericka McGowan, and Judy Estep.

PREFACE

Efforts to improve the safety and health of workers in the United States and around the world are vitally important. It is the committee's hope that this report can help move those efforts another step forward.

E. John Gallagher, *Chair*
Committee to Review the NIOSH Personal
Protective Technology Program

Contents

ABBREVIATIONS AND ACRONYMS — xvii

SUMMARY — 1

1 INTRODUCTION — 19
Scope of This Report, 20
Context and Background, 21
Overview of the NIOSH PPT Program, 24
Evaluation Approach, 30
Overview of This Report, 33
References, 33

2 RELEVANCE OF THE NIOSH PPT PROGRAM — 34
Overview of PPT Program Resources, 35
Goal 1: Reduce Exposures to Inhalation Hazards, 41
Goals 2 and 3: Reduce Exposures to Dermal and Injury Hazards, 63
Surveillance, 71
Overall Assessment of Relevance, 74
References, 76

3 IMPACT OF THE NIOSH PPT PROGRAM — 81
External Factors, 82

End Outcomes, 83
Intermediate Outcomes, 84
Overall Assessment of Impact, 97
References, 99

4 EMERGING ISSUES AND RESEARCH AREAS IN PERSONAL PROTECTIVE TECHNOLOGY   101
PPT Program's Process for Identifying Emerging Issues, 101
Committee's Assessment of the PPT Program's Process, 103
Emerging Issues Identified by the Committee, 104
References, 114

5 RECOMMENDATIONS FOR PPT PROGRAM IMPROVEMENT   116
Implement and Sustain a Comprehensive National PPT Program, 117
Establish PPT Research Centers of Excellence, 120
Enhance the Respirator Certification Process, 122
Increase Research on the Use and Usability of PPT, 125
Assess PPT Use and Effectiveness in the Workplace, 126
Concluding Remarks, 128
References, 129

APPENDIXES

A	Framework for the Review of Research Programs of the National Institute for Occupational Safety and Health	131
B	Methods: Committee Information Gathering	176
C	Information Provided by the NIOSH PPT Program	185
D	Biographical Sketches of Committee Members	187

Tables, Figures, and Boxes

TABLES

2-1 PPT Overall Budget Summary, 36
2-2 Breakdown of the PPT Program Budget by Objective, 38
2-3 Staff Allocations (FTE) by PPT Program Objectives, 39
2-4 Ongoing NIOSH Extramural Grants with a PPT Component, 41
2-5 Manufacturers' Respirator Certification Fees Retained by NIOSH, 43
2-6 Product Investigations, Including FFFIPP Investigations, 47
2-7 Number of Respirator Certifications by Category and Calendar Year, 48
2-8 Funding for NIOSH PPT Policy and Standards Development, 50
2-9 Steps in the Federal Rule-Making Process for Changes to 42 CFR 84, 52
2-10 Status of Federal Regulatory Changes (as of March 2008), 54

3-1 Recent Consensus Standards with PPT Program Involvement, 93

FIGURES

1-1 PPT-relevant efforts within the NIOSH organizational structure, 28
1-2 Logic model for the NIOSH Personal Protective Technology Program, 31

2-1 PPT Program funding by year and source, 35
2-2 PPT Program budget FY 2001-2007, 37

2-3   Funding sources for respirator certification by fiscal year, 42
2-4   Percentage of respirator certification applications processed within 90 days, 45

BOXES

S-1   PPT Program Strategic Goals and Objectives, 4
S-2   Scoring Criteria for Relevance, 7
S-3   Scoring Criteria for Impact, 9
S-4   Summary of Report Recommendations, 11

1-1   PPT Program Strategic Goals and Objectives, 26
1-2   NIOSH PPT Objectives Not Considered as Part of This Review, 27
1-3   Logic Model Terms and Examples, 32

2-1   NIOSH-Sponsored PPT Meetings, 51
2-2   Timeline of Key Events for the Dermal PPT Program—Inputs, Activities, and Outputs, 65
2-3   Scoring Criteria for Relevance, 76

3-1   Scoring Criteria for Impact, 98

Abbreviations and Acronyms

AIHA	American Industrial Hygiene Association
ANSI	American National Standards Institute
APR	air-purifying respirator
ASTM	originally, the American Society for Testing and Materials, now ASTM International
BLS	Bureau of Labor Statistics
CBRN	chemical, biological, radiological, and nuclear
CCSCBA	closed-circuit self-contained breathing apparatus
CDC	Centers for Disease Control and Prevention
CEL	Certified Equipment List
CFR	Code of Federal Regulations
COPPE	Committee on Personal Protective Equipment
CPIP	Certified Product Investigation Process
DHHS	Department of Health and Human Services
DHS	Department of Homeland Security
DoD	Department of Defense
DoL	Department of Labor
DRDS	Division of Respiratory Disease Studies (NIOSH)

EPA	Environmental Protection Agency
ERC	Education and Research Center (NIOSH)
ESLI	end-of-service-life indicator
FDA	Food and Drug Administration
FEV	forced expiratory volume
FFFIPP	Fire Fighter Fatality Investigation and Prevention Program
FTE	full-time equivalent
FVC	forced vital capacity
HEROES	Homeland Emergency Response Operational and Equipment Systems
HHE	Health Hazard Evaluation
IAB	InterAgency Board for Equipment Standardization and Interoperability
IAFF	International Association of Fire Fighters
IOM	Institute of Medicine
ISO	International Organization for Standardization
LTFE	Long-Term Field Evaluation
MINER Act	Mine Improvement and New Emergency Response Act of 2006
MOU	memorandum of understanding
MSHA	Mine Safety and Health Administration
NFPA	National Fire Protection Association
NIOSH	National Institute for Occupational Safety and Health
NIST	National Institute of Standards and Technology
NORA	National Occupational Research Agenda
NPPTL	National Personal Protective Technology Laboratory
NRC	National Research Council
OMB	Office of Management and Budget
OSHA	Occupational Safety and Health Administration
PAPR	powered air-purifying respirator
PASS	personal alert safety system
PPE	personal protective equipment
PPT	personal protective technology/technologies

r2p	research to practice
RKB	Responder Knowledge Base
SARS	severe acute respiratory syndrome
SCBA	self-contained breathing apparatus
SCSR	self-contained self-rescuer (respirator)
SEI	Safety Equipment Institute
SRUP	*Survey of Respirator Use and Practices*
TIL	total inward leakage
TSWG	Technical Support Working Group
UL	Underwriters Laboratories
USDA	U.S. Department of Agriculture

Summary

ABSTRACT *Protecting millions of workers from occupational hazards frequently involves the use of respirators, protective clothing, gloves, or other personal protective technologies (PPT). For some occupations, such as firefighting, the worker's protective equipment is the only form of protection against life-threatening hazards, while for others, such as healthcare workers, PPT is one component in a series of protective controls.*

In conjunction with a series of planned reviews of National Institute for Occupational Safety and Health (NIOSH) research programs, the Institute of Medicine (IOM) and the National Research Council (NRC) convened a committee of experts to review the NIOSH Personal Protective Technology Program (PPT Program) to evaluate the relevance of its work to improvements in occupational safety and health and the impact of its work in reducing workplace illnesses and injuries. Relevance was evaluated based on the priority of work carried out and the strength and plausibility of its association with improvements in workplace protection. Impact was evaluated based on contributions to intermediate and end outcomes linked to worker health and safety. The committee was also asked to assess the program's targeting of new research areas, identify emerging issues in PPT, and provide recommendations for strengthening the program. In addition to reviewing the PPT research efforts, the committee's task included evaluating the respirator certification program and appraising the policy and standards development efforts of the PPT Program.

Taking into account several important factors beyond the program's control, the committee found that since 2001 (the period covered by this review), the PPT Program has made meaningful contributions to improving worker health and safety. Using a five-point scoring scale (where 5 is highest), the committee assigned the NIOSH PPT Program a score of 4 for relevance. This score reflects the judgment that the PPT Program is working in priority areas and is engaged in transferring its research to improved products and processes. The committee also assigned the PPT Program a score of 4 for impact, indicating that the program has made probable contributions to end outcomes (improvements in worker health or safety) in addition to well-accepted intermediate outcomes.

To enhance the relevance and impact of its work, the committee recommends the development of a National PPT Program consistent with the original congressional mandate that would foster the development of improved protection for all workers through coordinated oversight of all PPT. The committee also recommends that the PPT Program establish research centers of excellence, enhance the respirator certification process, increase research on the use and usability of PPT, and assess PPT use and effectiveness in the workplace using a life-cycle approach.

OVERVIEW

Maintaining the health and safety of workers in the United States and globally is accomplished in part by reducing hazardous exposures through the use of personal protective equipment. Personal protective technologies (PPT) include respirators worn by construction workers and miners to protect against exposure to silica, dust, and hazardous gases; protective clothing, respirators, and gloves worn by firefighters and mine rescue workers to avoid burns and smoke inhalation; and respirators and protective clothing worn by healthcare workers to prevent acquiring an infectious disease. An estimated 5 million workers are required to wear respirators in 1.3 million U.S. workplaces. For some occupations, such as firefighting, the worker's protective equipment is the only form of protection against life-threatening hazards; for other workers, PPT is a supplement to ventilation and other environmental, engineering, or administrative hazard controls.

In the United States, federal responsibility for civilian worker PPT is integral to the mission of the National Institute for Occupational Safety and Health (NIOSH). This report examines the NIOSH Personal Protective Technology Program (PPT Program) and specifically focuses on the relevance and impact of this program in reducing hazardous exposures and improving worker health and safety.

STUDY PROCESS

In September 2004, NIOSH requested that the National Academies conduct evaluation reviews of specific NIOSH programs to assess the relevance and the impact of the work of NIOSH in reducing workplace injury and illness. For consistency across the set of evaluations, each evaluation review is using a methodology and framework developed by the National Academies' Committee to Review NIOSH Research Programs. In July 2007 the Institute of Medicine and the Division on Earth and Life Studies of the National Research Council formed the Committee to Review the NIOSH Personal Protective Technology Program. The committee included members with expertise in occupational health, emergency response, health care, personal protective equipment manufacturing, employee organizations, respiratory protection, dermal protection, injury protection, and program evaluation.

The committee was tasked with reviewing the NIOSH PPT Program and evaluating the program's relevance to and impact on occupational health and safety. In addition to reviewing PPT-related research programs, the committee's task included evaluating the certification and the standards development efforts of the PPT Program. Further, the committee was tasked with focusing its efforts on PPT relevant to respiratory and dermal hazards (Box S-1) as NIOSH efforts relevant to other types of PPT (e.g., hearing loss, fall prevention) are being addressed in other National Academies' reviews. The study committee was given the discretion to determine the time period to be covered by the review and chose to focus its evaluation from the inception of the NIOSH National Personal Protective Technology Laboratory (NPPTL) in 2001 through 2007.

THE NIOSH PPT PROGRAM

Personal protective technologies are defined as the specialized clothing or equipment worn by individuals for protection against health and safety hazards, as well as the technical methods, processes, techniques, tools, and materials that support their development, evaluation, and use. PPT encompasses personal protective equipment products such as respirators, gloves, protective eyewear, hearing protection, and protective clothing but also includes facepieces, filters, guidance documents, standards, and test procedures.

NIOSH's PPT Program works to fulfill its mission through three major areas of endeavor: (1) respirator certification as mandated in federal regulations; (2) research focused on protection from respiratory, dermal, and injury hazards; and (3) participation in standards setting and policy making. Workplaces regulated by the Occupational Safety and Health Administration (OSHA) or the Mine Safety and Health Administration (MSHA) in the United States with hazardous respiratory

BOX S-1
PPT Program Strategic Goals and Objectives

Strategic Goal 1: Reduce Exposure to Inhalation Hazards

Objective 1. Ensure the integrity of the national inventory of respirators through the implementation of a just-in-time respirator certification process.
Objective 2. Develop CBRN respirator standards to reduce exposure to CBRN threats.
Objective 3. Ensure the availability of mine emergency respirators for escape from mines.
Objective 4. Improve reliability and level of protection by developing criteria that influence personal protective equipment designs to better fit the range of facial dimensions of respirator users in the U.S. workforce.
Objective 5. Quantify the impacts of various personal protective equipment on viral transmission.
Objective 6. Evaluate the nanofiber-based fabrics and NIOSH-certified respirators for respiratory protection against nanoparticles.
Objective 7. Develop and make available end-of-service-life indicator (ESLI) technologies that reliably sense or model performance to ensure respirator users receive effective respiratory protection.
Objective 8. Gather information on the use of respirators in the workplace to identify research, intervention, and outreach needs.

Strategic Goal 2: Reduce Exposure to Dermal Hazards

Objective 1. Improve chemical-barrier protective clothing testing and use practices to reduce worker exposure to chemical dermal hazards.
Objective 2. Improve emergency responder protective clothing to reduce exposure to thermal, biological, and chemical dermal hazards.
Objective 3. Investigate physiological and ergonomic impact of protective ensembles on individual wearers in affecting worker exposure to dermal hazards.

Strategic Goal 3: Reduce Exposure to Injury Hazards*

Objective 1. Develop and evaluate warning devices for fire services.

NOTE: CBRN = chemical, biological, radiological, and nuclear.
*The PPT Program has additional objectives under this strategic goal that are related to hearing protection, protection from falls, and antivibration technologies. These objectives are not the focus of this review; some aspects of these objectives have been discussed in other National Academies' reviews.

exposures must meet federal requirements to provide their workers with NIOSH-certified respirators.[1] To achieve NIOSH certification, manufacturers submit respirator products to NPPTL, where the products undergo a series of certification tests depending on the type of respirator and its intended use. Products that successfully meet the design, quality, and performance certification criteria are designated and approved as NIOSH-certified respirators. Intramural research is conducted primarily in the more than 20 laboratory facilities located in Bruceton, Pennsylvania, near Pittsburgh. In addition, research is conducted through contracts with universities and other partners. The NIOSH extramural research program is administered through the NIOSH Office of Extramural Programs and is largely separate from the intramural program. The PPT Program's research portfolio is focused on respiratory research relevant to PPT, with a smaller but growing component of research on protective clothing and other types of PPT. NIOSH's work in PPT also involves participating in the development of relevant regulatory standards and consensus standards. Consensus standards for the manufacturing, performance, and testing of PPT products are developed by national and international standards development organizations. These organizations work through expert committees consisting of representatives from government agencies, manufacturers, employers, academia, and end users.

ASSESSMENT OF RELEVANCE

In considering the relevance of the PPT Program's efforts, the committee examined 12 of the program's objectives across the three principal domains of research, respirator certification, and policy and standards setting. The committee took into account the major external factors, particularly the limited budget and the regulatory mandate for respirator certification. Approximately one-third of the PPT Program's budget is designated for federally mandated respirator certification testing. The PPT Program operates in a set of multiple, small, partly refurbished laboratories dispersed over several acres. These facilities are inadequate for the challenges of overseeing the development of state-of-the-art PPT that must protect the health and safety of the nation's workers.

The respirator certification program is a premier function of the PPT Program. Since 2001, more than 1,600 respirators have been certified and substantive progress is being made in meeting the congressional mandate of completing certification within 90 days. However, having a long-standing spotlight on respirators, compounded by budget limitations, constrains efforts to address other types

---

[1] The Mine Safety and Health Administration (MSHA) is also involved in certifying certain mine escape equipment, and the Department of Defense has criteria specific to PPT for the military workforce.

of PPT (e.g., protective clothing, eye protection). Recent efforts, particularly in consensus standards setting, seem to be appropriately broadening the scope of the PPT Program.

NIOSH is one of only a few federal agencies that has onsite certification testing responsibilities and facilities. Because OSHA and MSHA require employers to purchase only NIOSH-certified respirators, NIOSH certification is viewed by manufacturers and employers as a business necessity. NIOSH certification regulations are in use by other countries as a model or basis for their respirator certification efforts. The PPT Program conducts a limited number of product audits and conducts manufacturer site audits using both staff and external consultants. Efforts to ensure the effectiveness of respirators would be strengthened through increased resources that could be directed toward field testing and expedited revision of the federal certification regulations.

The PPT Program has had well-documented success in its quick turnaround in developing the chemical, biological, radiological, and nuclear (CBRN) federal respirator standards. This effort involved extensive collaborative efforts with other federal agencies, nonprofit organizations, manufacturers, and others. The PPT Program is in the midst of updating regulations regarding the certification of mine self-rescue respirators. The PPT Program has conducted relevant research on total inward leakage, which is a major concern in respiratory protection, and on issues focused on criteria for powered air-purifying respirator regulations. However, the regulatory standards related to these issues are still in the initial stages of the rulemaking process, and expedited efforts are needed to move the process forward.

Consensus standards-setting activities are another priority area for the PPT Program and one in which it has been active through the technical committees that are highly relevant to the program's work. Participation in the development of ASTM (formerly, American Society for Testing and Materials) International, NFPA (National Fire Protection Association), and ISO (International Organization for Standardization) standards and test methods has been the primary mechanism for the PPT Program's productive engagement in standards designed to reduce hazardous dermal exposures. PPT Program research has also contributed to test methods and performance standards for protective gear.

The PPT Program is proactive in obtaining input from a range of stakeholders through a series of public meetings and manufacturers' meetings focused on specific topics or proposed changes to the certification regulations. Website and listserv capabilities are utilized for dissemination of invitations to upcoming public meetings, user notices, the Certified Equipment List, guidelines, and other key information. In the last few years, the PPT Program has become active in collaborations with various federal agencies and other partners and has begun to explore links with extramural researchers. As discussed in its recommendations, the committee urges a concentrated effort to bring the breadth of expertise in the extramural research community to bear on intramural and other pertinent PPT research questions.

The time frame for the committee's review began with the inception of the NPPTL in 2001. In this relatively short period of time, the program has initiated a range of relevant research projects. Some of the projects are the result of opportunities driven by external factors and funding, while others have been initiated by PPT Program investigators. Recent research initiatives have focused on PPT for pandemic influenza, and others have focused on efforts to examine the as-yet largely unknown implications of exposure to the products and by-products of nanotechnology. In addition to research to support and improve the respirator certification program (e.g., total inward leakage, anthropometrics), the committee suggests that the PPT Program address research in priority areas, particularly those for mining emergencies, dermal protection, and heat-related hazards. Limitations in the research budget are a major impediment to further improvements in PPT ensembles and in work that is needed across a range of occupations (e.g., agriculture, industry, construction, health care). While research has focused on engineering aspects of PPT, one of the challenges to be addressed in the near future is improving and ensuring usability. This will require particular emphasis on increasing safety by improving the comfort, wearability, and individual and organizational incentives needed to ensure that workers do in fact wear PPT.

On the basis of its review of the PPT Program's work in research, certification, and policy and standards setting, the committee has assigned the NIOSH Personal Protective Technology Program a score of 4 for relevance (Box S-2). This

---

BOX S-2
Scoring Criteria for Relevance

5 = The program's work is in high-priority subject areas, and NIOSH is significantly engaged in appropriate transfer activities for completed projects or reported results.
4 = The program's work is in priority subject areas, and NIOSH is engaged in appropriate transfer activities for completed projects or reported results.
3 = The program's work is in high-priority or priority subject areas, but NIOSH is not engaged in appropriate transfer activities; or the focus is on lesser priorities, but NIOSH is engaged in appropriate transfer activities.
2 = The program is focused on lesser priorities, and NIOSH is not engaged in or planning some appropriate transfer activities.
1 = The program is not focused on priorities, and NIOSH is not engaged in transfer activities.

score reflects the judgment that the PPT Program is working in priority areas and is engaged in transferring its research into improved products and processes. In the judgment of the committee, the program, with additional resources and an expanded focus, could further improve its relevance score by strengthening the product and site audit programs; expediting revisions to the federal regulatory standards; better harnessing the capabilities of the extramural research community; and placing a stronger emphasis on comfort, wearability, and other human factors that affect workers' use of PPT.

ASSESSMENT OF IMPACT

NIOSH is nationally and internationally recognized for its respirator certification program. OSHA and MSHA require that the respirators used in U.S. workplaces be NIOSH-certified. The PPT Program also took a leadership role in developing and expediting federal regulatory standards for CBRN respirators. This effort involved extensive collaboration with multiple federal agencies, manufacturers, and professional associations. For example, OSHA and NIOSH collaboratively developed a CBRN PPT Selection Matrix for Emergency Responders.

Impacts on reducing hazardous exposures or preventing illness or injury are difficult to attribute directly to the work of a single federal agency. However, because the PPT Program certifies that respirators meet a number of rigorous, prespecified performance criteria, the committee felt justified in acknowledging that positive end outcomes have occurred that are attributable to the PPT Program's role in respirator certification. For workers who have few other protections from hazardous workplace exposures, such as firefighters, the value of effective PPT is a daily reality. As noted above, successful mine escapes have occurred because the miners had access to effective respirators that prevented exposure to lethal levels of carbon monoxide. Having such equipment in place involves the collaborative efforts of manufacturers, professional associations, employers, employees, unions, state and federal agencies, and many others. However, the committee recognizes the central and vital role that the PPT Program plays in this effort.

Important intermediate outcomes also appear to be the result of active participation by PPT Program staff members in consensus standards-development efforts. The PPT Program has leveraged its limited resources well in its participation in national and international consensus standards organizations. Several recent ISO and ASTM International standards have incorporated test methods developed through PPT Program research. The PPT Program staff has also led or been instrumental in research on a number of key issues, although, as in several other important areas, budget restraints substantially limit the extent of research efforts. Work on protection against viral transmission (particularly related to pandemic influenza) and on nanotechnology is in the early phase and has not yet received the resources or had the opportunity to produce intermediate outcomes.

The committee believes that although great strides have been made in improving respirators, much could be done to address other types of PPT (e.g., protective clothing, protective eyewear, gloves, hearing protection, hard hats, fall harnesses) with additional resources. Additionally, the successful focus on improving PPT for emergency responders now needs to be expanded to other occupations, including agricultural workers, construction workers, healthcare workers, and industrial workers, where the public health impact is likely to be far more substantial. Work on protective ensembles also holds great promise, and innovative approaches need to be developed to provide seamless interfaces among different types and components of PPT.

The committee urges expedited efforts to revise federal certification regulations, so that new technologies and testing methodologies can be utilized to improve the efficacy of respirators and allow for innovation in the design and function of this equipment. Similarly, there is much that should be done to improve protective clothing, eyewear, gloves, and other types of PPT, contingent upon additional resources.

On the basis of its review of the PPT Program's work in research, respirator certification, and policy and standards setting, the committee has assigned the NIOSH Personal Protective Technology Program a score of 4 for impact. This score, according to the scoring criteria outlined by the framework committee, reflects the judgment that the PPT Program has made probable contributions to end outcomes in addition to well-accepted intermediate outcomes (Box S-3). In the judgment of the committee, the program could further improve its impact score

---

BOX S-3
Scoring Criteria for Impact

5 = The program has made major contribution(s) to worker health and safety on the basis of end outcomes or well-accepted intermediate outcomes.
4 = The program has made some contributions to end outcomes or well-accepted intermediate outcomes.
3 = The program's activities are ongoing, and outputs are produced that are likely to result in improvements in worker health and safety (with explanation of why not rated higher). Well-accepted outcomes have not been recorded.
2 = The program's activities are ongoing, and outputs are produced that may result in new knowledge or technology, but only limited application is expected. Well-accepted outcomes have not been recorded.
1 = Activities and outputs do not result in or are NOT likely to have any application.

by applying the lessons learned in the development of CBRN respirator standards to other types of PPT (e.g., protective clothing, protective eyewear, gloves) and emphasizing development and testing of protective ensembles and other integrated approaches to PPT.

EMERGING AREAS

In addition to examining the relevance and impact of the work of the NIOSH PPT Program, the committee was asked to examine the process by which the program identifies new research areas and to provide ideas on additional topics. The committee recognizes the many inputs to the PPT Program's process for establishing research priorities. The PPT Program sets its research and other institutional priorities through an ongoing strategic planning process that culminates in an annual planning summit attended by the governance team comprised of key PPT Program managers. Inputs to the planning process include the many public and manufacturers' meetings sponsored by the PPT Program that have recently been expanded to focus on a broader range of PPT efforts including hearing loss and fall prevention. The PPT Program has been very successful in engaging specific and familiar stakeholder groups, including respirator manufacturers and the emergency response community, and recognizes the need to expand into other work sectors. The PPT Program has demonstrated its engagement in PPT policy development through participation in consensus standards development committees and through its interactions with other federal agencies.

The PPT Program's process for identifying and addressing emerging areas seems quite open and transparent, and the committee urges the program to continue in this manner as it reaches out to other workplace sectors. The PPT Program would also benefit from further expertise in behavioral sciences and interdisciplinary specialties, aimed principally at human factors. Given the ongoing challenges of workers' noncompliance with PPT use, it is paramount that NIOSH recognize psychosocial, usability, comfort, and behavioral issues that profoundly modify the relationship between PPT design and user compliance.

The committee was not given the task of conducting a comprehensive assessment of all emerging issues in PPT, but it did identify several overarching considerations pertinent to all types of PPT: new materials technologies, usability and human factors, PPT ensembles and systems integration, enhancing a culture of workplace safety, and training and professional education.

RECOMMENDATIONS

The NIOSH PPT Program has made effective use of its limited resources and has moved the research, standards-setting, and certification agendas forward, largely with a focus on respirators. However, much still has not been done due to serious budgetary constraints. The committee offers the following recommendations (Box S-4) with the goal of improving the ability of the NIOSH PPT Program to broaden its scope and depth of responsibility in order to protect workers more effectively from hazardous workplace exposures, illness, injuries, and disease.

BOX S-4
Summary of Report Recommendations

Recommendation 1: Implement and Sustain a Comprehensive National Personal Protective Technology Program

NIOSH should work to ensure the implementation of the 2001 congressional mandate for a comprehensive state-of-the-art federal program focused on personal protective technology. A comprehensive program would build on the current NIOSH PPT Program and would bring unified responsibility and oversight to all PPT-related activity at NIOSH.

Recommendation 2: Establish PPT Research Centers of Excellence and Increase Extramural PPT Research

The PPT Program should establish and sustain extramural PPT centers of excellence and work to increase other extramural research opportunities.

Recommendation 3: Enhance the Respirator Certification Process

The PPT Program should continue to improve the respirator certification process. The program should expedite the revision of the respirator certification regulations, develop a mechanism for registering the purchase of NIOSH-certified respirators, expand the product audit program, monitor the site audit program, and disseminate respirator certification test result data.

Recommendation 4: Increase Research on the Use and Usability of PPT

The PPT Program should intensify its research directed at barriers to and facilitators of PPT use by workers. Such research should examine human factors and ergonomics, as well as individual behaviors and organizational behaviors, particularly workplace safety culture.

Recommendation 5: Assess PPT Use and Effectiveness in the Workplace Using a Life-Cycle Approach

The PPT Program, in collaboration with relevant NIOSH divisions and other partners, should oversee an ongoing surveillance and field testing program to assess PPT use and effectiveness in the workplace. These efforts should emphasize a life-cycle approach by including both pre-market and interval post-market testing of PPT and include data collection on issues ranging from training to decontamination.

Recommendation 1: Implement and Sustain a Comprehensive National Personal Protective Technology Program

NIOSH should work to ensure the implementation of the 2001 congressional mandate for a comprehensive state-of-the-art federal program focused on personal protective technology. A comprehensive program would build on the current NIOSH PPT Program and would bring unified responsibility and oversight to all PPT-related activity at NIOSH. The National Personal Protective Technology Program should

- Oversee, coordinate, and where appropriate, conduct research across all types of occupational PPT and across all relevant occupations and workplaces;
- Participate in policy development and standards setting across all types of occupational PPT;
- Oversee all PPT certification in order to ensure a minimum uniform standard of protection and wearability. The National Program should collaborate with other relevant government agencies, private-sector organizations, and not-for-profit organizations to conduct an assessment of the certification mechanisms needed to ensure the efficacy of all types of PPT; and
- Promote the development, standards setting, and certification of effectively integrated PPT components and ensembles in which multiple types of PPT (e.g., eye protection, hearing protection, respirators) can be effectively and seamlessly worn together.

The committee was struck by the discordance between the congressional mandate[2] to establish the National Personal Protective Technology Laboratory (NPPTL) in 2001 and the challenges faced by the current PPT Program, which focuses almost solely on respiratory PPT because of limited resources. If NIOSH is to respond fully to its 2001 congressional directive to develop and test state-of-the-art national PPT needs (respirators, protective clothing, gloves, hearing protection, eye protection, and other types of PPT) across all relevant work sectors, then a more comprehensive approach is needed.

---

[2]Senate Report 106-293 stated "It has been brought to the Committee's attention the need for design, testing and state-of-the-art equipment for this nation's 50 million miners, firefighters, healthcare, agricultural and industrial workers. . . . The Committee encourages NIOSH to carry out research, testing and related activities aimed at protecting workers, who respond to public health needs in the event of a terrorist incident. The Committee encourages CDC [the Centers for Disease Control and Prevention] to organize and implement a national personal protective equipment laboratory."

As PPT becomes increasingly complex, integration of its many components requires scrupulously coordinated development of interfaces and ensembles that are designed, standardized, and certified under the oversight of a single entity within NIOSH, dedicated solely to PPT in the workplace. To promote worker safety by integrating various types of protective equipment requires placing the responsibility for all PPT efforts at NIOSH under a single entity that has the responsibility and the requisite resources to oversee the broad array of PPT and to lead the efforts to provide workers with improved and innovative protective equipment.

In 2005, NIOSH took a significant first step toward coordinating PPT-related efforts across the institute by establishing the PPT Program and developing a matrix approach to management. However, the committee is concerned that the current matrix structure of PPT efforts at NIOSH is too ambiguously configured to serve the long-term needs and flexible goals of a comprehensive, coordinated national PPT endeavor. Although designated as a program in name, the directors of the current PPT Program have limited budgetary authority and management responsibility for PPT research and other efforts outside of NPPTL. As a result of the lack of a single authority there are major gaps in integration, coordination, and consolidation of many types of PPT. The current matrix approach, while a good first step, does not bring the full depth and range of NIOSH expertise to bear on moving forward in improving and coordinating PPT at the national level.

The committee believes that a meaningfully integrated approach to improving all types of occupational PPT would logically require consolidation of the oversight responsibilities for PPT efforts at NIOSH. The committee's emphasis in response to its charge was on proposing a general strategy intended to optimize the wealth of relevant expertise at NIOSH in order to meet the new challenges of developing fully integrated and coordinated protective ensembles and technologies for worker protection. Approaches could range from maintaining current laboratory and research facilities with changes in reporting and budgetary authority to more major organizational changes. Carrying out the original congressional intent of an effort focused on "the design, testing, and state-of-the-art [personal protective] equipment for this nation's . . . workers" (Senate Report 106-293) will necessitate a commitment to a broad scope of work and collaborative efforts.

Recommendation 2: Establish PPT Research Centers of Excellence and Increase Extramural PPT Research

The PPT Program should establish and sustain extramural PPT centers of excellence and work to increase other extramural research opportunities. The PPT Program should

- **Develop and support research centers of excellence that work closely with the NIOSH intramural research program to improve PPT, increase field research, and explore and implement research to practice interventions; and**
- **Work with the NIOSH Office of Extramural Programs to increase other research opportunities and enhance collaboration and awareness of relevant PPT research efforts among intramural and extramural researchers.**

The community of extramural scientists is a highly valuable resource for improving PPT. It is critical that this breadth and depth of expertise is focused on important PPT research questions relevant to improving PPT and to transferring PPT research into workplace practice. Successful efforts to address critical issues in many other fields of scientific inquiry have been the result of investing in extramural research centers of excellence. Research centers of excellence allow for interdisciplinary expertise and improved ability to evaluate interventions such as new technologies, while facilitating strong collaborations. Increased intramural research resources and personnel, extramural grants, cooperative agreements, and direct contracts should be balanced to leverage PPT capabilities. Where feasible, the PPT Program should take advantage of existing expertise, laboratory infrastructure, and outreach networks, which may be costly to duplicate in the intramural PPT Program. In addition to expanding the resources dedicated to PPT research and development, a strong extramural community provides the opportunity to extend scientific inquiry into the behavioral sciences and other types of expertise that might not be available within the NIOSH PPT Program. PPT centers of excellence should be aligned with one or more of the scientific focus areas of the PPT Program. The centers could be developed to be topic-specific (e.g., heat stress, dermal permeation) or to be sector-specific to explore the unique PPT needs of a particular occupation or set of workers. Several types of centers would be optimal. University-based research centers could establish collaborative networks with other universities and with nonprofit organizations and federal agencies focused on research and development of innovative approaches to PPT. Complementary centers of excellence would be those that are centered in nonprofit organizations, state departments of health or labor, or agencies with capabilities and expertise in post-market or field research. These centers, in conjunction with partner organizations and universities, could increase field research, and explore and implement research to practice interventions. Multi-year funding and evaluation are critical to build a strong and ever-improving research base.

Recommendation 3: Enhance the Respirator Certification Process

The PPT Program should continue to improve the respirator certification process. The program should

- Expedite the revision of the respirator certification regulations. As a part of that effort, NIOSH should revise the respirator certification fee schedules so that certification fees paid by respirator manufacturers fully cover the cost of certification. NIOSH's research budget for PPT research should not be eroded by the costs of certification.
- Develop a mechanism for registering the purchase of NIOSH-certified respirators so that post-marketing notifications and recalls can be accomplished expeditiously and effectively.
- Expand the audit programs to ensure that results of the product audit program are methodologically and statistically sound and that the site audit program ensures standardized quality of audits whether performed by NIOSH staff or contractors.
- Disseminate respirator certification test result data (e.g., breathing resistance).

Respirator certification has been a significant part of the work of the PPT Program. In FY 2007, almost half (approximately 48 percent) of the PPT Program's $13.1 million budget was designated for the certification program (in prior years, certification generally constituted about a third of the program's total budget). In FY 2007, certification occupied about half of the PPT Program's full-time equivalent workforce. The NIOSH respirator certification process is highly respected and provides a major contribution to worker safety. The committee believes that although the enhancements to the certification program recommended above will require additional resources, the dividends that will accrue to workers from improved standards, audits, and information dissemination will make such an investment sustainable and well worth the start-up costs.

Improving respirators, and thereby reducing exposures to respiratory hazards, is in large part an effort focused on updating, refining, and developing the tests and performance criteria that respirators must meet to provide effective protection in the workplace. These tests are specified through federal regulations, many of which have not been changed significantly in more than 35 years. The PPT Program through NPPTL has developed a modular approach to updating federal regulations. The committee sees these revisions and additions to the regulatory standards as a major opportunity for the PPT Program to improve respirators through updated tests that address current and evolving technologies. An issue of concern to the committee was the extent of federal resources devoted to the costs of respirator certification, costs that would more appropriately be borne by respirator manufacturers as is done for other types of product certification.

Recommendation 4: Increase Research on the Use and Usability of PPT

The PPT Program should intensify its research directed at barriers to and facilitators of PPT use by workers. Such research should examine human factors and ergonomics, as well as individual behaviors and organizational behaviors, particularly workplace safety culture.

One of the greatest challenges to PPT effectiveness is ensuring that the worker is wearing the equipment and is wearing it correctly. Understanding that comfort is fundamentally a *safety* issue is a necessary prerequisite to improvement of the materials, design, and engineering of PPT in such a way that critically important human factors are taken into account. Improving usability will require research that focuses on task- and worker-centered design and a more in-depth knowledge of physiologic burdens (often heat stress) resulting from wearing PPT in the work environment. The PPT Program is moving forward in its work with the National Fire Protection Association and other partners in addressing these issues, particularly as they relate to physiologic burdens for emergency responders and firefighters. However, similar efforts are needed to assess usability issues for the majority of the workforce employed in other occupations.

Recommendation 5: Assess PPT Use and Effectiveness in the Workplace Using a Life-Cycle Approach

The PPT Program, in collaboration with relevant NIOSH divisions and other partners, should oversee an ongoing surveillance and field testing program to assess PPT use and effectiveness in the workplace. These efforts should emphasize a life-cycle approach by including both pre-market and interval post-market testing of PPT and include data collection on issues ranging from training to decontamination. Enhanced efforts would

- **Assess and critically appraise PPT use and effectiveness across all types of PPT (e.g., gloves, eye protection, respirators) and across relevant industry sectors and workplace environments;**
- **Require random periodic field testing of an adequately sized sample of PPT to assess effectiveness, usability, and durability with reasonable accuracy and precision; and**

- **Build on existing government and private-sector surveys and surveillance activities that collect PPT-relevant data and facilitate linkages to other datasets.**

Improvements in PPT will be driven both by efficacy data generated in the laboratory and effectiveness data gathered with equal scientific rigor in the workplace. Research priorities for PPT should be based on the prevalence and degree of exposure, modified by the strength of the observed association between these attributes of exposure and long- and short-term outcomes of illness and injury. The committee urges the NIOSH PPT Program to assess the effectiveness and use of PPT in the workplace across all phases of the lifetime of the products. This type of evaluation and surveillance construct could involve an array of approaches and methodologies, including pre- and post-market field testing of PPT products, surveys, on-site observations, focus groups and other end user inputs, as well as outcome and impact evaluations and formal cost-benefit analysis. Obtaining input from the end user of PPT products is particularly important.

In considering how best to plan and learn from a life-cycle approach to data collection that will involve field testing and ongoing surveillance, it will be important to keep in mind that the immediate goals will differ with pre- and post-market field testing focused on the effectiveness of a specific product and surveillance focused on an ongoing assessment of PPT use. The committee believes these efforts are a necessary and vital investment for improving PPT and protecting workers from hazardous exposures. By choosing the appropriate methodologies and by building on current data collection efforts, sound investments can be made in obtaining data that are representative of workplace use and useful in improving PPT products and training.

CONCLUDING REMARKS

The committee urges NIOSH to reexamine its commitment to PPT with a focus that is directly proportional to its importance to the safety and health of millions of workers in the many workplaces where administrative and engineering controls are inadequate, impractical, or simply nonexistent.

NIOSH's Personal Protective Technology Program has made significant strides in improving PPT available to workers, especially respiratory PPT. It is the committee's hope that the recommendations in this report will provide the necessary impetus for the development of a National Personal Protective Technology Program that conducts, coordinates, and provides national oversight of research, standards setting, and certification for all components of PPT and the interface between and among those components. The committee concludes, on the basis of all available evidence, that increasing the protection of workers from hazardous workplace exposures through the development and deployment of improved personal protective technologies is not only a critically important and worthwhile goal for workers in the United States and around the world but, with additional resources and thoughtful reorganization, is by no means out of reach.

1

Introduction

Protecting the health and safety of workers in the United States and globally is accomplished in part by reducing hazardous exposures through the use of personal protective equipment and other protective technologies. Personal protective technologies (PPT) include respirators worn by construction workers and miners to protect against exposure to silica, dust, and hazardous gases; protective clothing, respirators, and gloves worn by firefighters and mine rescue teams to avoid burns and smoke inhalation; and respirators and protective clothing worn by healthcare workers to prevent acquiring an infectious disease. An estimated 5 million workers are required to wear respirators in 1.3 million U.S. workplaces (OSHA, 2007b). For some occupations, such as firefighting, the worker's protective equipment is the only form of protection against life-threatening hazards; for other workers, PPT is a supplement to ventilation and other environmental, engineering, or administrative hazard controls.

In the United States, federal responsibility for civilian worker PPT is integral to the mission of the National Institute for Occupational Safety and Health (NIOSH). This report examines the NIOSH Personal Protective Technology Program (PPT Program) and specifically focuses on the relevance and impact of this program in reducing hazardous exposures and improving worker health and safety. The report also identifies important emerging issues in the future of PPT and closes with recommendations targeted at enhancing personal protective technologies for all workers.

SCOPE OF THIS REPORT

In September 2004, NIOSH requested that the National Academies conduct evaluation reviews of specific NIOSH programs to assess the relevance and the impact of the work of NIOSH in reducing workplace injury and illness. Further, NIOSH requested that each evaluation study committee be asked to assess and identify emerging research issues for that program and to provide recommendations for program improvement. In response, a set of evaluation studies is being conducted by ad hoc committees of the Institute of Medicine (IOM) and the National Research Council (NRC). Each committee evaluation is using a similar methodology and framework (Appendix A) developed by the National Academies' Committee to Review NIOSH Research Programs. The framework aims to provide a consistent format across the set of evaluation studies.

The Personal Protective Technology Program was one of the programs selected by NIOSH to be included in this series of reviews. In July 2007 the Institute of Medicine and the Division on Earth and Life Studies of the National Research Council formed the Committee to Review the NIOSH Personal Protective Technology Program. The committee included members with expertise in occupational health, emergency response, health care, personal protective equipment manufacturing, employee organizations, respiratory protection, dermal protection, injury protection, and program evaluation.

The committee was tasked with reviewing the NIOSH PPT Program and evaluating the program's relevance to and impact on occupational health and safety. The task of this committee was slightly modified in comparison with the other evaluation committees, so that it included the charge to review the respirator certification program and the standards development efforts of the PPT Program, in addition to reviewing the PPT-related research programs.

Specifically the committee was asked to provide the following:

- Assessments of the program's contribution[1] to reductions in workplace hazardous exposures, illnesses, or injuries through
  - an assessment of the relevance of the program's activities to the improvement of occupational safety and health, and
  - an evaluation of the impact that the program has had in reducing work-related hazardous exposures, illnesses, and injuries

---

[1] Because of the addition of the certification and standards elements of the PPT Program, this evaluation also considers additional outcomes such as adoption of new technologies and changes in knowledge, attitudes, and behaviors.

- A rating of the performance of the PPT Program for its relevance and impact using an integer score of 1 to 5: Impact could be assessed directly (e.g., reductions in illnesses or injuries) or, as necessary, using intermediate outcomes to estimate impact (qualitative narrative evaluations are included to explain the numerical ratings)
- Assessments of the program's effectiveness in targeting new research areas, activities, outputs, and outcomes and identification of emerging issues that the program should be prepared to address
- Recommendations for program improvement

As explained in more detail later in this chapter, the committee was tasked with focusing its efforts on PPT relevant to respiratory and dermal hazards. The study committee was given the discretion to determine the time period to be covered by the review and chose to focus its evaluation from the inception of the National Personal Protective Technology Laboratory (NPPTL) in 2001 through 2007.

The committee held three meetings from September 2007 to March 2008, of which two included open sessions in which the PPT Program was discussed with NIOSH staff, PPT manufacturers, representatives from professional associations and labor unions, and other stakeholders (Appendix B). Additionally, in November 2007, committee members participated in a site visit to the PPT Program's facilities in Pittsburgh, Pennsylvania.

CONTEXT AND BACKGROUND[2]

Personal protective technologies are defined as the specialized clothing or equipment worn by individuals for protection against health and safety hazards, as well as the technical methods, processes, techniques, tools, and materials that support their development, evaluation, and use (OSHA, 2002; NIOSH, 2007b). PPT encompasses personal protective equipment products such as respirators, gloves, protective eyewear, hearing protection, and protective clothing but also includes facepieces, straps, service life indicators, filters, guidance documents, standards, and test procedures.

The brief overview of PPT provided below describes the context of PPT within other occupational safety and health efforts and also highlights the roles of federal agencies and other organizations involved in PPT.

---

[2]This section draws on text from the 2008 Institute of Medicine report *Preparing for an Influenza Pandemic: Personal Protective Equipment for Healthcare Workers.*

PPT and Occupational Safety and Health

PPT is an essential component in the continuum of occupational safety and health efforts. Although PPT is generally considered as a last line of defense in the hierarchy of protective controls, it is important to note that in many jobs (e.g., firefighting), PPT is the only means available to protect workers from serious hazards. PPT is particularly vital for workers who must face hazards in emergency response situations, healthcare workers for protection from infectious agents where the environmental control remains largely undetermined (e.g., SARS, avian influenza), or those who work in outdoor environments or face other conditions in which the work environment is difficult to control (e.g., an influenza pandemic in which large numbers of patients would overwhelm the availability of isolation rooms).

In the traditional hierarchy of controls, process changes or substitution are optimal because they eliminate or reduce the hazard. Engineering and environmental controls (e.g., air exchanges, air filtration, negative-pressure rooms) that can isolate the hazard or reduce exposure or potential for injury are considered the next level of defense against hazardous exposures because they are measures that affect a large number of workers and patients and do not depend on individual compliance (Thorne et al., 2004). Administrative controls have been considered the third level of defense because the policies, standards, warnings, alarms, and procedures (including access restrictions, rotating workers to reduce individual exposures, and instilling a culture of workplace safety) established within an organization can substantially limit hazardous exposures and improve worker safety. Although PPT is often considered the last level of defense against hazardous exposures, its importance should not be minimized. The contribution to disease and injury prevention provided by each of these layers of exposure control (including PPT) is likely to vary considerably based on the specific tasks and local conditions.

It is also important to note that personal protective technologies are used by the general public in settings that range from hobbies to home-based businesses to protection against infectious disease. Many employers now provide safety and wellness messages and training for their workforce about being safe outside of work. Thus, the work being done by the NIOSH PPT Program has the potential to go well beyond the workplace.

Relevant Agencies and Organizations

The testing, regulation, and use of PPT involve a number of government and nongovernmental agencies and organizations. In the federal government, civilian occupational health and safety is the responsibility of both the Department of Health and Human Services (DHHS) and the Department of Labor (DoL). The

INTRODUCTION

Occupational Safety and Health Act of 1970 created two federal agencies to address worker safety and health: NIOSH (in DHHS) was designated with responsibilities for relevant research, training, and education, and OSHA (the Occupational Safety and Health Administration in DoL) was designated with responsibilities for developing and enforcing workplace safety and health regulations. NIOSH tests and certifies respirators and conducts and funds research in PPT. NIOSH also plays an integral role in relevant standards setting for many types of PPT (see further details later in this chapter and in Chapter 2).

OSHA regulates the use of PPT products in most U.S. workplaces. Respirators used by workers in OSHA- and MSHA (Mine Safety and Health Administration)-regulated workplaces must be certified by NIOSH to meet specific effectiveness criteria. Further, OSHA respirator regulations (29 CFR 1910.134) detail employer responsibilities for establishing and maintaining a comprehensive respiratory protection program, including requirements for performance of a risk assessment to select the proper respirator; annual training; and a program of inspection, cleaning, and disinfection. OSHA also has a general regulatory standard (29 CFR 1910.132) and related regulations for the maritime, construction, and mining industries that govern all other forms of PPT. The federal Occupational Safety and Health Act of 1970 encourages states to develop and operate their own job safety and health programs. Currently, 22 states and jurisdictions operate plans that cover both private-sector and state and local government employees, while 4 states and jurisdictions cover public employees only (OSHA, 2007a).

Other departments, agencies, and organizations also have a role in testing and improving PPT. MSHA is actively involved in testing and developing PPT in conjunction with NIOSH for mining applications. The Department of Defense develops and tests PPT for military applications. The Department of Homeland Security focuses on emergency response PPT and works to coordinate and improve standards and equipment-related issues. The Environmental Protection Agency addresses PPT issues relevant to pesticide exposures and emergency response readiness. The Consumer Product Safety Commission has oversight responsibilities for PPT products sold in the commercial marketplace. The Food and Drug Administration (in DHHS) has federal regulatory authority to provide manufacturers with the approval or clearance to market personal protective devices used in health care. PPT products that claim to provide protection against a specific health hazard must have FDA approval or market clearance. For any other PPT products sold in the commercial marketplace, there are no requirements stipulating pre-market or other testing prior to their sale to the public. For those products that assert NIOSH certification, NIOSH has the authority to act against mislabeled products.

Federal agencies, PPT manufacturers, employers, and others utilize testing methods and performance requirements for PPT that are based on consensus standards developed by standards-development organizations such as the International Organization for Standardization.

OVERVIEW OF THE NIOSH PPT PROGRAM

The PPT Program is 1 of 24 cross-sector programs at NIOSH. Developed in conjunction with the National Occupational Research Agenda (NORA), the NIOSH Program Portfolio is organized both by specific occupational sectors (e.g., construction, manufacturing, mining) and by issues and entities that cut across work sites (e.g., emergency preparedness and response, global collaborations, personal protective technology, hearing loss prevention). The PPT Program's mission is to "prevent work-related injury, illness, and death by advancing the state of knowledge and application of personal protective technologies" (NIOSH, 2007a). The program's vision statement follows (NIOSH, 2007a):

> The vision is to be the leading provider of quality, relevant, and timely PPT research, training, and evaluation. PPT in this context is defined as the technical methods, processes, techniques, tools, and materials that support the development and use of personal protective equipment worn by individuals to reduce the effects of their exposure to a hazard.

The PPT Program encompasses the PPT-relevant work conducted within several NIOSH divisions that addresses occupational protection against respiratory, dermal, and injury hazards. The NIOSH intramural activities related to PPT to reduce respiratory and dermal hazards are performed primarily within the National Personal Protective Technology Laboratory (NPPTL) (Figure 1-1). Ongoing research in the Division of Respiratory Disease Studies intersects with the inhalation-related research, and work in the Dermal Exposure Research Program interconnects with dermal-related PPT research at NPPTL. Intramural efforts on PPT involved in injury prevention (e.g., hearing loss, fall prevention, antivibration) are performed in the Division of Safety Research, Pittsburgh Research Laboratory, the Division of Applied Research and Technology, and the Health Effects Laboratory Division. In addition, the PPT Program, like other cross-sector NIOSH programs, is supported by efforts of the Education and Information Division; the Division of Surveillance, Hazard Evaluations, and Field Studies; the Office of Extramural Programs; and the Health Effects Laboratory Division.

Because of the cross-sector and interdisciplinary nature of PPT efforts, the NIOSH PPT Program, established in 2005, has been administered through a matrix management structure that aims to integrate PPT efforts and to implement a collaborative and cohesive research and policy agenda. Under this matrix structure, the

NPPTL director is the responsible manager for the PPT Program and the NPPTL associate director for science is the coordinator for all of the related research activities. The NIOSH cross-sector program alignment in 2005 was the impetus for the development of the PPT Program's matrix structure (NIOSH, 2007b).

The PPT Program has identified three strategic goals:

1. Reduce exposure to inhalation hazards.
2. Reduce exposure to dermal hazards.
3. Reduce exposure to injury hazards.

The first two goals are the focus of efforts at NPPTL, while the work on injury hazards is more widely dispersed across several NIOSH divisions. Each of these goals has been further subdivided into a set of objectives determined through the PPT Program's strategic planning process.

The committee was asked to focus on strategic goals 1 and 2 encompassing inhalation and dermal hazards[3] (Box 1-1). Most of the PPT Program objectives related to injury hazards (strategic goal 3) have been examined to some extent by other National Academies' reviews including the report on the hearing loss research program (IOM and NRC, 2006) and the forthcoming report on the traumatic injury research program. The committee needed to use consistent terminology throughout this report and decided to use the term "PPT Program" to denote the efforts from the inception of NPPTL in 2001 to the present that have been conducted by NIOSH relevant to the 12 PPT objectives that the committee was tasked with examining (Box 1-1). The objectives listed in Box 1-2 include PPT research related to hearing loss, falls, and hand vibration. These efforts are being conducted in several NIOSH divisions (see Figure 1-1) but are not examined in detail in this report because, as noted above, they are addressed in other National Academies' reviews.

PPT Program Efforts

The NIOSH PPT Program works to fulfill its mission through three major areas of endeavor: (1) respirator certification, (2) research, and (3) participation in standards setting and policy making. These efforts are interrelated, but each requires appropriate resources and partnering initiatives to be effective.

As mentioned above, OSHA- and MSHA-regulated workplaces in the United States with hazardous respiratory exposures must meet federal requirements to

---

[3]One objective related to strategic goal 3 on warning devices for firefighters was also included in the committee's purview.

**BOX 1-1
PPT Program
Strategic Goals and Objectives**

Strategic Goal 1: Reduce Exposure to Inhalation Hazards

Objective 1. Ensure the integrity of the national inventory of respirators through the implementation of a just-in-time respirator certification process.
Objective 2. Develop CBRN respirator standards to reduce exposure to CBRN threats.
Objective 3. Ensure the availability of mine emergency respirators for escape from mines.
Objective 4. Improve reliability and level of protection by developing criteria that influence personal protective equipment designs to better fit the range of facial dimensions of respirator users in the U.S. workforce.
Objective 5. Quantify the impacts of various personal protective equipment on viral transmission.
Objective 6. Evaluate the nanofiber-based fabrics and NIOSH-certified respirators for respiratory protection against nanoparticles.
Objective 7. Develop and make available end-of-service-life indicator (ESLI) technologies that reliably sense or model performance to ensure respirator users receive effective respiratory protection.
Objective 8. Gather information on the use of respirators in the workplace to identify research, intervention, and outreach needs.

Strategic Goal 2: Reduce Exposure to Dermal Hazards

Objective 1. Improve chemical-barrier protective clothing testing and use practices to reduce worker exposure to chemical dermal hazards.
Objective 2. Improve emergency responder protective clothing to reduce exposure to thermal, biological, and chemical dermal hazards.
Objective 3. Investigate physiological and ergonomic impact of protective ensembles on individual wearers in affecting worker exposure to dermal hazards.

Strategic Goal 3: Reduce Exposure to Injury Hazards

Objective 1. Develop and evaluate warning devices for fire services.

NOTE: CBRN = chemical, biological, radiological, and nuclear.
*The PPT Program has additional objectives under this strategic goal that are related to hearing protection, protection from falls, and antivibration technologies (Box 1-2). These objectives are not the focus of this review; some aspects of these objectives have been discussed in other National Academies' reviews.

INTRODUCTION

> **BOX 1-2**
> **NIOSH PPT Objectives Not Considered as Part of This Review**
>
> **Strategic Goal 3: Reduce Exposure to Injury Hazards**
>
> Objective 2. Develop measurement and rating methods that are representative of the real-world performance of hearing protection devices.
> Objective 3. Develop hearing protection laboratory and fit testing methods.
> Objective 4. Evaluate the effectiveness of hearing protection devices to provide protection from impulsive noise.
> Objective 5. Develop an integrated hearing protection and communication system.
> Objective 6. Develop hearing protection recommendations for noise-exposed hearing-impaired workers.
> Objective 7. Develop and improve fall arrest harnesses.
> Objective 8. Select and develop vibration isolation devices to reduce hand-arm vibration syndrome.

provide their workers with NIOSH-certified respirators.[4] To achieve NIOSH certification, manufacturers submit respirator products to NPPTL, where the products undergo a series of certification tests depending on the type of respirator and its intended use (NIOSH, 2007c). Products that successfully meet the design, quality, and performance certification criteria are designated and approved as NIOSH-certified respirators. Federal regulations for NIOSH certification of respirators are outlined in detail in the Code of Federal Regulations (42 CFR Part 84), and any changes to the certification criteria must comply with the federal rule-making process.

The PPT Program encompasses both intramural and extramural research components. Intramural research is conducted primarily in the more than 20 laboratory facilities located in Bruceton, Pennsylvania, near Pittsburgh. In addition, research is conducted through contracts with universities and other partners. The NIOSH extramural research program is administered through the NIOSH Office of Extramural Programs and is largely separate from the influence of the intramural program. As described in Chapters 2 and 3, the PPT Program's research portfolio is focused on PPT for respiratory protection, with a smaller but growing component of research on protective clothing and other types of PPT.

---

[4]The Mine Safety and Health Administration (MSHA) is also involved in certifying certain mine escape equipment, and the Department of Defense has criteria specific to PPT for the military workforce.

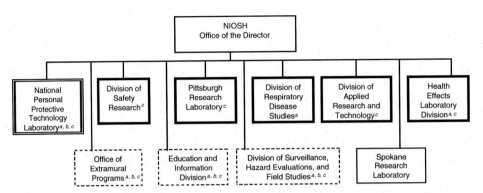

FIGURE 1-1 PPT-relevant efforts within the NIOSH organizational structure. In 2005, NIOSH organized its portfolio into programmatic categories that represent industry sectors and cross-sector programs organized around adverse health outcomes, statutory programs, and global efforts. The PPT Program is a cross-sector program that crosses most organizational units. For the scope of this report, the PPT Program is defined as the work conducted at NPPTL since 2001 related to the 12 objectives described in Box 1-1. Additional units conducting PPT-relevant research are indicated by bolded borders. Units supporting PPT Program activities are indicated by dashed borders. The Office of Extramural Programs funds PPT research grants managed by extramural grant recipients. The Education and Information Division translates PPT research findings to scientific information products for dissemination to the workplace. The Division of Surveillance, Hazard Evaluations, and Field Studies conducts workplace investigations to inform the workplace of PPT guidance and regulations and to obtain information on occupational exposures where standards are lacking or do not protect all workers. The Spokane Research Laboratory is not currently conducting any PPT-related efforts.
NOTE: [a]Unit conducts PPT-related efforts relevant to inhalation hazards.
[b]Unit conducts PPT-related efforts relevant to dermal hazards.
[c]Unit conducts PPT-related efforts relevant to injury hazards.

NIOSH's work in PPT also involves participating in the development of relevant regulatory standards and consensus standards. Consensus standards for the manufacturing, performance, and testing of PPT products are developed by national and international standards development organizations. These organizations work through expert committees consisting of representatives from government agencies, manufacturers, employers, academia, and end users. PPT Program staff members are involved in efforts of the International Organization for Standardization (ISO); ASTM International (formerly, American Society for Testing and Materials); the American National Standards Institute (ANSI); and the National Fire Protection Association (NFPA).

History of the PPT Program

Efforts by the U.S. government relevant to PPT can be traced back to work by the U.S. Bureau of Mines, which was created in 1910. The Bureau of Mines developed a program of respirator research, performance testing, and analysis and served as the certifying agency for respirators until NIOSH was established in 1971 (NIOSH, 2007b).

In the early 1970s, NIOSH and the Bureau of Mines worked jointly to codify the requirements and processes for respirator certification and testing (30 CFR Part 11[12]). In 1972, NIOSH was designated with primary responsibility for the performance testing of respirators. Additionally, NIOSH developed a PPT research program that began to focus on PPT issues relevant to a range of workers including those employed in mining and agricultural work (NIOSH, 2007b). Researchers also assessed the potential use of military gas masks for workplace applications. Prior to 1995, all respirator certifications were issued jointly by MSHA and NIOSH using 30 CFR Part 11 regulations. In 1995, new respirator certification regulations (42 CFR Part 84) were adopted, and NIOSH became the sole approving authority for most respirators.[5] When the U.S. Bureau of Mines was abolished in the mid-1990s, the Pittsburgh Research Laboratory, including its hearing protection research work, was transferred to NIOSH. Respirator certification was housed within the Division of Safety Research through the mid-1990s when it was transferred to the Division of Respiratory Disease Studies. One of the influential efforts in setting PPT research priorities in the first decade of the National Occupational Research Agenda was a 1998 workshop sponsored by NIOSH, the American Industrial Hygiene Association, and the American Society of Safety Engineers.

In 2001, a congressional mandate to expand NIOSH's occupational safety and health research included a directive for NIOSH to establish a National Personal Protective Technology Laboratory. The congressional intent, as outlined in Senate Report 106-293, stated that

> [i]t has been brought to the Committee's attention the need for design, testing and state-of-the-art equipment for this nation's 50 million miners, firefighters, healthcare, agricultural and industrial workers. . . . The Committee encourages NIOSH to carry out research, testing and related activities aimed at protecting workers, who respond to public health needs in the event of a terrorist incident. The Committee encourages CDC [the Centers for Disease Control and Prevention] to organize and implement a national personal protective equipment laboratory.

Early efforts at NPPTL, particularly in FY 2001 and FY 2002, were focused on renovating laboratory and office facilities at Bruceton. Respirator certification was transferred from the Division of Respiratory Disease Studies to NPPTL. Additional

---

[5]Specific mine emergency devices are certified jointly by NIOSH and MSHA.

PPT-related efforts, including PPT for chemical and biological hazards and life support and disaster response, were also transferred to NPPTL. PPT efforts related to reducing exposure to injury hazards (fall harnesses, vibration gloves, hearing protection) remained dispersed across other NIOSH divisions. Most recently in 2005, under the NIOSH cross-sector program alignment, the PPT Program was established. Initial efforts of the PPT Program focused on identifying all PPT-related activities in NIOSH.

EVALUATION APPROACH

Like other IOM and NRC committees that were charged with reviewing the major NIOSH programs (IOM and NRC, 2006; NRC and IOM, 2007, 2008a,b), the committee followed the guidance of the framework developed by the National Academies' Committee to Review NIOSH Research Programs (Appendix A). This set of guidelines was used in evaluating the relevance of the program's work to improvements in occupational safety and health and in assessing the impact that NIOSH efforts have had in reducing workplace illnesses and injuries. The framework committee has suggested that relevance be evaluated in terms of the degree of research priority and connection to improvements in workplace protection. Factors taken into account include the frequency and severity of hazardous exposures, the size of the worker population at risk, the structure of the program, and the degree of consideration given to stakeholder input (see Appendix A). The impact of the program is to be evaluated in terms of its contributions to the end outcomes of worker health and safety and to intermediate outcomes that might reasonably be expected to contribute to reduction in illness and injury over time. The evaluation is to take the form of qualitative narrative assessments as well as the assignment of two integer scores between 1 and 5 for the relevance and impact of the Personal Protective Technology Program.

The guidance in the Framework Document reflects the terminology and organization of a logic model adopted by NIOSH to characterize the steps in its work. The logic model used by the PPT Program (Figure 1-2) reflects the many roles of the PPT Program, because it includes components related to respirator certification and standards setting as well as those related to research. An examination of goals, inputs, activities, and outputs was used to assess the relevance of the program. End outcomes and intermediate outcomes were the principal focus for the evaluation of the program's impact. External factors were taken into consideration in the evaluation. The terms used in the logic model are defined in Box 1-3.

The study charge also directs the committee to review the progress that the PPT Program has made in identifying new research and to provide additional ideas on emerging areas relevant to the program's mission (Chapter 4). According to the Framework Document, the committee's identification of emerging research areas

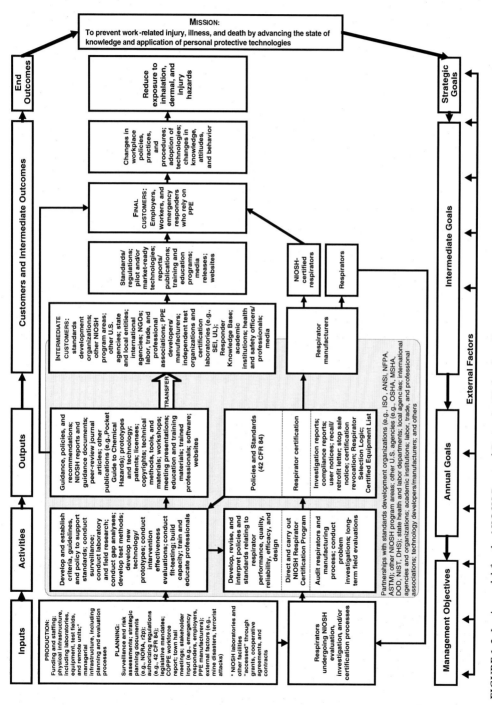

FIGURE 1-2 Logic model for the NIOSH Personal Protective Technology Program.
SOURCE: NIOSH, 2007b.

> **BOX 1-3**
> **Logic Model Terms and Examples**
>
> **Planning Inputs:** Stakeholder input, surveillance and intervention data, and risk assessments (e.g., input from Federal Advisory Committee Act panels or the National Occupational Research Agenda research partners, intramural surveillance information, Health Hazard Evaluations [HHEs]).
>
> **Production Inputs:** Intramural and extramural funding, staffing, management structure, and physical facilities.
>
> **Activities:** Efforts and work of the program, staff, grantees, and contractors (e.g., surveillance, health effects research, intervention research, health services research, information dissemination, training, technical assistance).
>
> **Outputs:** Direct products of NIOSH programs that are logically related to the achievement of desirable and intended outcomes (e.g., publications in peer-reviewed journals, recommendations, reports, website content, workshops and presentations, databases, educational materials, scales and methods, new technologies, patents, technical assistance).
>
> **Intermediate Outcomes:** Related to the program's association with behaviors and changes at individual, group, and organizational levels in the workplace. An assessment of the worth of NIOSH research and its products by outside stakeholders (e.g., production of standards or regulations based in whole or in part on NIOSH research; attendance at training and education programs sponsored by other organizations; use of publications, technologies, methods, or recommendations by workers, industry, and occupational safety and health professionals in the field; citations of NIOSH research by industry and academic scientists).
>
> **End Outcomes:** Improvements in safety and health in the workplace. Defined by measures of health and safety and of impact on processes and programs (e.g., changes related to health, including decreases in injuries, illnesses, or deaths and decreases in exposures due to research in a specific program or subprogram).
>
> **External Factors:** Actions or forces beyond NIOSH's control (e.g., by industry, labor, regulators, and other entities) with important bearing on the incorporation in the workplace of NIOSH's outputs to enhance health and safety.
>
> SOURCE: Adapted from IOM and NRC, 2006.

is to be done using members' expert judgment rather than a formal research needs assessment. The committee was also charged with providing recommendations for improving the PPT Program (Chapter 5).

OVERVIEW OF THIS REPORT

The committee provides its assessment of the NIOSH PPT Program in the remaining chapters of this report. Chapter 2 discusses the program's budget, staffing, other production and planning inputs, activities, and outputs and presents the committee's assessment and rating of the program's relevance to the priorities of work in PPT. In Chapter 3, the committee examines the intermediate and end outcomes that could reasonably be attributed to the work of the PPT Program and provides its rating of the program's impact in reducing injury and illness among workers. Chapter 4 reviews the program's mechanisms for identifying emerging issues and highlights some additional considerations that in the view of the committee warrant future attention. The report concludes in Chapter 5 with the committee's recommendations for strengthening the PPT Program and increasing its relevance to, and impact on, health and safety in the workplace.

REFERENCES

IOM (Institute of Medicine). 2008. *Preparing for an influenza pandemic: Personal protective equipment for health care workers.* Washington, DC: The National Academies Press.

IOM and NRC (National Research Council). 2006. *Hearing loss research at NIOSH.* Committee to Review the NIOSH Hearing Loss Research Program. Rpt. No. 1, Reviews of Research Programs of the National Institute for Occupational Safety and Health. Washington, DC: The National Academies Press.

NIOSH (National Institute for Occupational Safety and Health). 2007a. *Personal Protective Technology Program.* http://www.cdc.gov/niosh/programs/ppt/ (accessed March 19, 2008).

NIOSH. 2007b. *NIOSH Personal Protective Technology Program: Evidence for the National Academies Committee to Review the NIOSH Personal Protective Technology Program.* Pittsburgh, PA: NIOSH.

NIOSH. 2007c. *NPPTL topic: Respirator testing.* http://www.cdc.gov/niosh/npptl/stps/respirator_testing.htm (accessed March 19, 2008).

NRC and IOM. 2007. *Mining safety and health research at NIOSH.* Committee to Review the NIOSH Mining Safety and Health Research Program. Rpt. No. 2, Reviews of Research Programs of the National Institute for Occupational Safety and Health. Washington, DC: The National Academies Press.

NRC and IOM. 2008a. *Agriculture, forestry, and fishing research at NIOSH.* Committee to Review the NIOSH Agriculture, Forestry, and Fishing Research Program. Rpt. No. 3, Reviews of Research Programs of the National Institute for Occupational Safety and Health. Washington, DC: The National Academies Press.

NRC and IOM. 2008b. *Respiratory disease research at NIOSH.* Committee to Review the NIOSH Respiratory Disease Research Program. Rpt. No. 4, Reviews of Research Programs of the National Institute for Occupational Safety and Health. Washington, DC: The National Academies Press.

2

Relevance of the NIOSH PPT Program

The committee began its assessment of the relevance of the Personal Protective Technology (PPT) Program of the National Institute for Occupational Safety and Health (NIOSH) by looking at the resources available to the program, the decisions and priorities set by the program, and the products and other outputs and transfer activities that have resulted from the efforts of the PPT Program since 2001.[1] This chapter begins with an overview of the program's current resources and interactions, followed by a detailed analysis of the relevance of the PPT Program's efforts in addressing its goals of reducing exposures to inhalation, dermal, and injury hazards through PPT. The chapter concludes with a summary assessment of the relevance of the PPT Program.

As discussed in Chapter 1, the committee was asked to assess the work of the NIOSH PPT Program relevant to 12 objectives. Other National Academies' reports (IOM and NRC, 2006; NRC and IOM, 2007, 2008a,b) have examined NIOSH programs on hearing loss, mining, and respiratory disease, which encompass related PPT elements. Additional National Academies' reports on NIOSH's construction, traumatic injury, and health hazard evaluation programs will also be relevant.

---

[1] As defined in Chapter 1, this report uses the term *PPT Program* to refer to the efforts from 2001 to the present that have been conducted by NIOSH relevant to the 12 PPT-relevant objectives that focus primarily on protection against respiratory and dermal hazards (Box 1-1).

OVERVIEW OF PPT PROGRAM RESOURCES

Funding and Staffing

Since its initial funding in FY 2001, the PPT Program's annual budget has ranged from $8.6 million to $12.2 million with additional funding sources adding between $1.3 million and $8.8 million (Figure 2-1). These figures do not encompass PPT-relevant work on hearing loss, fall protection, and antivibration gloves. Extramural research funding is provided through the NIOSH Office of Extramural Programs (see below).

The PPT Program's funding from external sources, which totaled $1.3 million in FY 2007 but was as high as $8.8 million in FY 2003, has been largely targeted at PPT for first responders in the event of a terrorist attack. These activities also included the development and implementation of federal regulations to certify respirators designed to reduce exposures to chemical, biological, radiological, and nuclear (CBRN) hazards. Sources of external funding for this project included the National Institute of Standards and Technology (NIST), the Department of Homeland Security, and the U.S. Department of the Navy. In recent years, both external funding and the PPT Program's budget have simultaneously declined (Figure 2-1; Table 2-1).

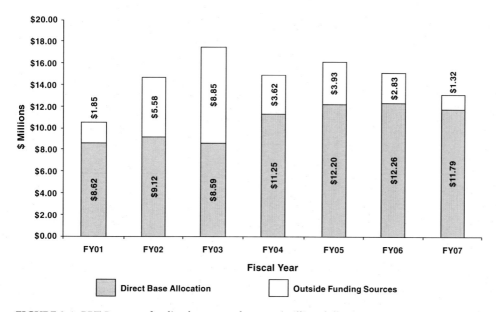

FIGURE 2-1 PPT Program funding by year and source (million dollars).
SOURCE: NIOSH, 2007a.

TABLE 2-1 PPT Overall Budget Summary

	FY 2001	FY 2002	FY 2003	FY 2004	FY 2005	FY 2006	FY 2007	FY 2008	Total
Direct budget allocation	$8,616,297	$9,116,297	$8,593,373	$11,248,770	$12,200,070	$12,259,922	$11,787,202	$11,779,970	$85,601,901
External funding	$1,847,519	$5,576,000	$8,850,760	$3,616,139	$3,933,314	$2,826,992	$1,317,002	$148,094	$28,115,820
Total	$10,463,816	$14,692,297	$17,444,133	$14,864,909	$16,133,384	$15,086,914	$13,104,204	$11,928,064	$113,717,721

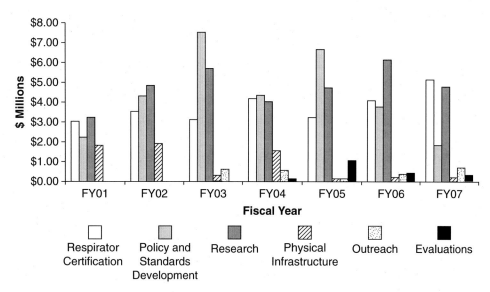

FIGURE 2-2 PPT Program budget FY 2001-2007.
SOURCE: NIOSH, 2007a.

To gain further insights into the allocation of the funding resources, the committee also examined annual funding levels by objective and by use (Table 2-2 and Figure 2-2). In the first three years of the National Personal Protective Technology Laboratory (NPPTL) (FY 2001 to FY 2003), significant resources were needed to renovate the laboratory and office space. Recent changes have allocated increased resources for outreach and for evaluation.

Several segments of the PPT Program budget are dedicated to specific activities (NIOSH, 2007a). Evaluation efforts (e.g., National Academies' evaluations, peer reviews, customer satisfaction surveys) are protected activities addressing issues relevant to all areas of the research, standards-setting, and certification efforts. Similarly, the PPT Program dedicates resources to its research-to-practice (r2p) activities[2] to ensure that the results of its scientific activities in the laboratory can be translated into efforts to improve workplace safety.

Initial staffing in the first year NPPTL was created included 19 full-time equivalent (FTE) personnel from existing NIOSH divisions and 11 competitive hires from other government agencies, academia, and private industry. By FY 2007, PPT Program staffing stood at 61 FTE federal employees (Table 2-3). The distribution of the expertise of the FTE positions at NIOSH emphasizes the applied science

---

[2] A NIOSH initiative focused on the transfer and translation of research findings, technologies, and information into effective prevention practices and products that can be adopted in the workplace.

TABLE 2-2 Breakdown of the PPT Program Budget by Objective

PPT Program Objective	FY 2001	FY 2002	FY 2003	FY 2004	FY 2005	FY 2006	FY 2007	FY 2008	Total	Percentage
Dermal Objectives										
Protective clothing tests	$778,074	$747,360	$493,294	$688,051	$746,998	$638,186	$198,683	$153,852	$4,444,498	3.9
Emergency responders	$0	$0	$0	$0	$290,950	$182,584	$203,225	$96,828	$773,587	0.7
Physiological impact	$0	$496,403	$1,273,489	$600,373	$683,919	$992,351	$740,412	$947,738	$5,734,685	5.0
Injury Objective										
PASS warning devices	$720,987	$318,529	$503,517	$324,497	$546,519	$113,243	$176,453	$69,681	$2,773,426	2.4
Inhalation Objectives										
Certification	$3,095,419	$3,797,557	$2,316,706	$5,186,286	$4,340,557	$4,570,614	$6,392,211	$5,845,022	$35,544,372	31.3
CBRN	$2,873,300	$6,084,128	$10,401,677	$5,282,899	$6,411,547	$4,411,428	$1,258,337	$1,612,456	$38,335,772	33.7
Mining	$1,464,746	$1,007,911	$697,199	$949,245	$447,403	$235,194	$1,681,040	$602,256	$7,084,994	6.2
Anthropometrics and TIL	$1,012,158	$676,597	$513,880	$381,632	$1,277,875	$600,014	$291,964	$781,938	$5,536,058	4.9
Viral transmission	$0	$0	$0	$0	$0	$1,463,738	$777,552	$481,139	$2,722,429	2.4
Nanotechnology	$0	$0	$0	$0	$0	$310,175	$325,351	$319,111	$954,637	0.8
ESLI	$0	$1,323,477	$931,980	$1,131,645	$1,120,658	$1,294,696	$688,003	$620,891	$7,111,350	6.3
Surveillance	$519,131	$240,335	$312,390	$320,283	$266,959	$274,690	$370,974	$397,154	$2,701,916	2.4
Total	$10,463,815	$14,692,297	$17,444,132	$14,864,911	$16,133,385	$15,086,913	$13,104,205	$11,928,066	$113,717,724	100.0

NOTE: ESLI = end-of-service-life indicator; PASS = personal alert safety system; TIL = total inward leakage.
This table breaks down the PPT Program's annual budget by program objective. Overarching costs are spread across all goals by percentage. Overarching costs include funding for the Office of the Director; personnel, services and benefits; Quality of Science initiatives (National Academies reviews, IOM standing committee); APEX (Achieving Performance Excellence) activities; and outreach activities. For example, in this table the 31.3 percent of the budget allocated for certification activities includes 31.3 percent of the overarching costs described above.
SOURCE: NIOSH, 2008d.

TABLE 2-3 Staff Allocations (FTE) by PPT Program Objectives

Objectives	FY 2001	FY 2002	FY 2003	FY 2004	FY 2005	FY 2006	FY 2007	FY 2008	Total
Dermal Objectives									
Protective clothing tests	3.20	4.19	3.24	3.21	2.52	1.52	1.10	0.85	19.83
Emergency responders	0.00	0.00	0.00	0.00	0.30	0.56	1.85	0.45	3.16
Physiological impact	0.00	0.36	1.14	1.75	3.45	2.51	1.04	3.26	13.51
Total	3.20	4.55	4.38	4.96	6.27	4.59	3.99	4.56	36.50
Injury Objective									
PASS warning devices	0.09	0.67	0.75	1.22	1.32	0.75	0.86	0.61	6.27
Inhalation Objectives									
Certification	14.48	24.35	21.56	26.46	31.49	29.33	33.13	38.03	218.83
CBRN	13.32	15.03	16.59	13.70	18.81	13.90	7.84	11.54	110.73
Mining	4.54	6.52	4.35	4.64	1.88	1.50	4.23	3.61	31.27
Anthropometrics and TIL	1.46	3.90	3.80	2.26	3.57	3.99	1.75	3.41	24.14
Viral transmission	0.00	0.00	0.00	0.00	0.00	1.20	4.32	3.42	8.94
Nanotechnology	0.00	0.00	0.00	0.00	0.00	1.23	1.19	1.02	3.44
ESLI	0.00	1.18	1.46	1.75	2.45	1.78	2.04	2.00	12.66
Surveillance	0.97	1.27	2.06	2.19	1.63	1.72	2.07	2.13	14.04
Total	34.77	52.25	49.82	51.00	59.83	54.65	56.57	65.16	424.05
PPT Program Total	38.06	57.47	54.95	57.18	67.42	59.99	61.42	70.33	466.82

NOTE: ESLI = end-of-service-life indicator; PASS = personal alert safety system; TIL = total inward leakage.
SOURCE: NIOSH, 2008e.

nature of the work. In FY 2007, the FTE positions were primarily in the engineering, physical sciences, and quality assurance fields. The PPT Program has one full-time epidemiologist on staff. NIOSH staff members in other offices and divisions can collaborate on PPT Program projects.

Facilities

The PPT Program is administered through NPPTL, with the main campus located outside of Pittsburgh, Pennsylvania, at the Bruceton Research Facility. At the Bruceton location, the PPT Program's work is spread throughout 26 laboratories and testing facilities. These facilities include climatic chambers, flammability and vibration testing machines, an anthropometrics research laboratory, and a recently added human research physiology laboratory. A recent renovation expanded the fit test laboratory to allow for total inward leakage (TIL) assessment as a part of quantitative fit testing.

The current laboratories are housed in renovated buildings. In 2002, soon after NPPTL was established, a development study was undertaken to explore the needs and costs of developing the laboratory and administrative space needed to fulfill the congressional mandate for the PPT Program. The goals of the consolidation effort were to "improve communication among researchers, centralize related projects, and thus improve program efficiency" (Jacobs Facilities, 2002). The development study explored program and space requirements. In 2002, the total costs of building and implementing an approximately 122,700 square foot facility were estimated at $91 million (Jacobs Facilities, 2002). An update of the development plan was conducted in 2006. Unfortunately, the original concept of a unified laboratory with modern space has not been realized, and the current configuration of the disparate laboratories largely isolates researchers from each other and is counterproductive to collaborative research efforts.

The facilities that house the work of some of the other PPT components in NIOSH include auditory research laboratories in Pittsburgh and in Cincinnati, Ohio; an anthropometry laboratory that examines the ergonomic performance of safety equipment and industrial tools in Morgantown, West Virginia; and a human performance research laboratory at Pittsburgh Research Laboratory.

Extramural Research

The NIOSH Office of Extramural Programs administers the investigator-initiated extramural program. Grant applications are reviewed through scientific review groups (study sections) managed by scientific review administrators at NIOSH or in the Center for Scientific Review at the National Institutes of Health

(NIOSH, 2008l). Of the nine identified extramural projects with ongoing work relevant to PPT, two grants support work in agricultural safety and health centers and one supports work on construction safety (Table 2-4). PPT Program staff reported that they are working to develop an improved strategy for using the output of the extramural research program as input to the planning and priority-setting processes of the relevant components of the PPT Program (NIOSH, 2007a).

Efforts to more fully engage the extramural research community are needed. A variety of options exist including research centers of excellence (Chapter 5), cooperative agreements, small business innovation research (SBIR) programs, and small business technology transfer (STTR) programs. The PPT Program should take as active role a role as possible in developing extramural research and encouraging these researchers to explore innovative approaches to improving PPT.

GOAL 1: REDUCE EXPOSURES TO INHALATION HAZARDS

Respirator Certification

A major factor in reducing worker exposure to inhalation hazards is ensuring that respirators effectively protect the user. Respirator certification is a congressionally mandated activity requiring NIOSH to certify respirators in accordance with 42 CFR Part 84. Under this regulation, NIOSH is responsible for directing and conducting laboratory, field, quality, and research functions related to respirator certification. Specifically, the PPT Program, through NPPTL, establishes certification testing criteria, conducts product testing, reviews the technical specifications for the product, and examines the manufacturer's quality assurance program. The PPT Program also performs product and site audits and evaluates product

TABLE 2-4 Ongoing NIOSH Extramural Grants with a PPT Component

Start and End Dates	Grant Title
9/2006 to 9/2011	Pacific Northwest Agricultural Safety and Health Center
9/2006 to 8/2011	Northeast Center for Agricultural Health
8/2006 to 7/2011	Active hearing protectors and audibility of critical communications
7/2005 to 7/2010	Respirator effects in impaired workers
8/2006 to 7/2009	Enclosing hood effectiveness
9/2004 to 6/2009	Centers for Construction Safety and Health
8/2006 to 7/2008	Measuring human fatigue with the BLT prototype
7/2005 to 6/2008	Assessment methods for nanoparticles in the workplace
4/2005 to 3/2008	Multipurpose protective clothing for emergency responders

SOURCE: NIOSH, 2007a.

complaints as a part of the certification process. In addition, the PPT Program conducts research focused on improving testing and evaluation methods. NIOSH has been responsible for administering the respirator certification program since 1972. NIOSH and the Mine Safety and Health Administration (MSHA) jointly certify mine emergency devices.

Planning and Production Inputs

Budgets Approximately 30 percent of the PPT Program's budget from 2001 through 2007 was allocated to the respirator certification program (Table 2-2). Funding for the certification program comes from two sources: federally appropriated funds and certification fees charged to manufacturers submitting a certification application. Since 2001, overall funding for the respirator certification program has ranged from approximately $2.3 million to $6.4 million (Table 2-2).

More than 90 percent of the funding for respirator certification is provided through federal funding (Figure 2-3; Table 2-5). The certification fee schedules for traditional respirators were set in 1972 and have not been revised since. Fees range from $750 for supplied-air respirators to $4,100 for gas masks and filtering self-rescuer respirators and from $100 to $900 for subcomponents (42 CFR Part 84). Additional fees can be levied if an examination, inspection, or testing procedure exceeds the normal level of effort; however, the additional fees are limited to a maximum of $100 "per man day expended." In 2002, NIOSH was authorized to

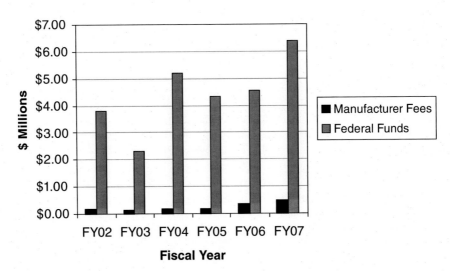

FIGURE 2-3 Funding sources for respirator certification by fiscal year.
SOURCE: NIOSH, 2007b.

TABLE 2-5 Manufacturers' Respirator Certification Fees Retained by NIOSH

Fees Retained by NIOSH	FY 2001	FY 2002	FY 2003	FY 2004	FY 2005	FY 2006	FY 2007
Non-CBRN respirators	0	$183,800	$104,450	$120,850	$140,000	$130,150	$280,990
CBRN respirators[a]	0	$7,000	$9,300	$53,200	$45,020	$196,842	$196,829
Total	0	$190,800	$113,750	$174,050	$185,020	$326,992	$477,819

[a]Funding of CBRN live agent testing is paid through NIOSH to the U.S. Army Research, Development, and Engineering Command. These funds are not included in the table.
SOURCE: NIOSH, 2007b.

retain the fees charged to manufacturers; prior to that time the fees were deposited in the general fund of the U.S. Treasury.

In FY 2007, the certification program's budget (including overhead) was approximately $6.39 million (Table 2-2). Of that amount, only $477,819 (approximately 8 percent) was covered by certification fees received from manufacturers (Table 2-5) (NIOSH, 2007b). To recover the actual costs of respirator certification efforts in FY 2007, NIOSH would have needed to increase its certification fees by 13 to 15 times the current amount.

When the new CBRN regulations were developed (discussed below), the fee structure for CBRN certification stipulated significantly higher certification fees due to the high costs of live agent testing. Fees for CBRN respirator certification range from $175 to $21,735 (NPPTL, 2007). Although the costs for the live agent testing are covered by these higher fees, the remainder of the costs for certification testing and processing by NIOSH are not fully covered by manufacturers.

The committee believes that the costs of certification testing should be borne by respirator manufacturers and that the fee structure for traditional respirators is in immediate need of revision. The fees have not been revised for more than 30 years while certification costs have increased steadily. The U.S. market for respiratory protection in 2003 was estimated at approximately $2 billion (Frost and Sullivan, 2005). An increase in fees could fully fund certification activities and allow the use of federal resources to increase research efforts to improve PPT and better protect the nation's workers (Chapter 5).

Staffing Implementing the respirator certification process is the responsibility of NPPTL's Technology Evaluation Branch, which in FY 2007 had 26 full-time employees. In FY 2007, management personnel consisted of a branch chief, two team leaders, and two technical analysts. Application processing requires two FTEs to conduct an initial review, two FTEs to review quality assurance, two FTEs to function as team leaders, and analysts to conduct the final review phase. Respirator testing is conducted by eight NIOSH FTEs and four contract employees. Additionally, two contract employees and one NIOSH FTE provide administrative support. It should be noted that while the PPT Program has the personnel, facilities, equipment, and procedures to perform this work with a high degree of quality, it does not have significant redundancy in either testing personnel or facilities, so that any temporary reduction in personnel or any equipment malfunction could delay certification work.

Activities

The PPT Program has a robust process for carrying out its federal mandate to test, evaluate, and certify respirators. The process involves application processing, respirator testing, and quality assurance plan evaluation; product and site audits; and respirator equipment evaluation.

Processing and respirator testing Respirator manufacturers submitting applications for certification must be registered with NIOSH and obtain a manufacturer's code to allow for evaluation of the manufacturer's quality assurance program. The NIOSH certification program currently has approximately 90 active approval holders with 100 manufacturing sites worldwide (NIOSH, 2007a). In the past five years, the certification program has processed approximately 1,900 applications (of which more than 1,400 were granted certification after testing and approximately 500 were rejected). Since 2001, over 1,600 respirator certification requests have been granted. In addition to submitting sample respirator units for testing, applications for respirator certification include results of pre-testing of the proposed design.

Sample respirators undergo a series of test procedures (depending on the category of respirator) that have been developed by NIOSH and specified in federal regulations. Tests conducted at the PPT Program's facilities include detailed evaluations of the efficacy of the filters, determination of exhalation valve leakage, and evaluations of breathing resistance as well as many other specific tests. Air-purifying elastomeric facepiece respirators are tested for facepiece fit by human test subjects. The test procedures are available online for use by manufacturers prior to certification submission (NIOSH, 2008m). In addition to laboratory tests of sample respirators, the PPT Program also evaluates the manufacturer's quality assurance program.

As part of its certification efforts, the PPT Program conducts research on improved testing and certification methodologies. Current research efforts include the enhancement of existing technology to support respirator certification (total inward leakage tests and a quality assurance module) and enhancements to standard test procedures. New standard test procedures are being developed to deal with innovative or novel technologies such as antimicrobial and adhesive technologies.

The goal for completion of the certification process is 90 days as stipulated by Congress (Senate Report 104-368). The PPT Program has made significant efforts to meet the 90-day goal. In 2007, 81 percent of applications for air-purifying and air-supplied respirator certification were processed within 90 days compared to 75 percent in 2003 (NIOSH, 2007c; Figure 2-4). Data for the total number of air-purifying and air-supplied respirators from 2003 to 2007 show that 76 percent of applications were processed by the PPT Program in 90 days or less.[3]

Product and site audits Audits are conducted to verify implementation and efficacy of quality control plans, which are evaluated as part of the certification requirements. Quality assurance evaluations are conducted via product and site audits. Issuance of respirator certification requires that manufacturers maintain quality facilities, processes, and products. Each manufacturing location undergoes a site audit every two years. Mine escape respirator manufacturers undergo yearly audits.

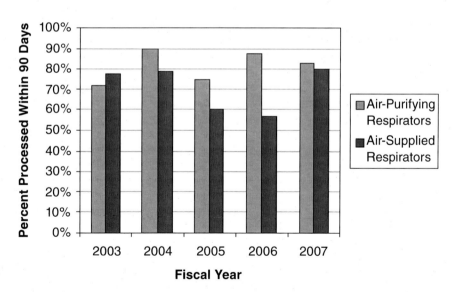

FIGURE 2-4 Percentage of respirator certification applications processed within 90 days.
SOURCE: NIOSH, 2007c.

---

[3]Percentage of applications processed within 90 days is based on the PPT Program turnaround days, which refers to the total number of days the application is available for processing within the PPT Program.

Since 2001, site audits have been conducted in 16 to 43 sites annually (NIOSH, 2007b). Contractors approved and hired by the PPT Program can conduct routine initial and follow-up site audits; non-routine audits, depending on their nature, may require direct involvement of NIOSH staff members. Information provided by the PPT Program detailed the costs of facility audits as $6,000 for U.S. manufacturing facilities and $12,000 for audits conducted outside the United States.

The PPT Program also conducts 40 to 60 product audits per year by selecting respirators from normal sales and distribution outlets and testing them to determine product quality (NIOSH, 2007a). The PPT Program realizes that this is not a statistically significant sample and, although constrained by limited resources, is working to expand its program. One specialized type of product audit conducted by the PPT Program is the Long-Term Field Evaluation (LTFE) program, which examines the performance of mine escape respirators using a sample of respirators collected from working mines. Deployed self-contained self-rescuers (SCSRs) are compared to new SCSRs using a series of selected tests that follow the certification test standards. The most recent phase of the evaluation program found that all deployed SCSRs show some evidence of performance degradation (NIOSH, 2006). The PPT Program is working to revise the LTFE program to enhance the statistical integrity of the sampling strategy (NIOSH, 2007f). Resources are fairly limited, with approximately $570,000 devoted to this effort in FY 2007 and about half of that in FY 2006 and FY 2005 (approximately $200,000 and $240,000, respectively) (NIOSH, 2008a). The committee strongly supports expanded activities in product and field testing to provide much-needed information on the life cycle of PPT equipment and the realities of work site performance (see Chapter 5).

Respirator equipment investigations The PPT Program investigates reports of problems with all NIOSH-certified respirators through its Certified Product Investigation Process (CPIP). These investigations can be prompted by user complaints, product evaluations, or the NIOSH Fire Fighter Fatality Investigation and Prevention Program (FFFIPP).[4] For product inquiries, the PPT Program's role is to validate the report through testing and to monitor corrective actions by the manufacturer (if needed). The PPT Program also provides technical assistance to the manufacturer as needed. If a problem is not addressed, NIOSH has the authority to require a manufacturer to recall or retrofit a product or to revoke certification. Since 2001, product investigations (not including FFFIPP investigations) have been opened on 220 products (Table 2-6). Information about the product investigation program and the mechanism for requesting an investigation are not

---

[4]The PPT Program is part of the NIOSH FFFIPP, which investigates deaths of firefighters in the line of duty with the goal of preventing future deaths and injuries (NIOSH, 2008p). The PPT Program is involved in tests of respirators and other protective equipment.

TABLE 2-6 Product Investigations, Including FFFIPP Investigations[a]

Fiscal Year	Product Investigations Opened (not including FFFIPP)	FFFIPP Investigations Opened	Total Closed
2007	9	3	10
2006	26	6	37
2005	36	2	65
2004	33	4	23
2003	31	8	31
2002	46	5	39
2001	39	5	43
Total	220	33	248

NOTE: FFFIPP = Fire Fighter Fatality Investigation and Prevention Program.
[a]Through August 17, 2007.
SOURCE: NIOSH, 2007a.

readily apparent on the NIOSH website. The committee urges efforts to provide additional web-based information including a contact point, as well as other efforts to inform employers and respirator users regarding how to submit issues needing investigation.

Outputs

The most significant output of the respirator certification program is the number of respirator certifications issued, thereby increasing the potential inventory of certified respirators available to workers. Since 2001 the PPT Program has issued more than 1,600 respirator certifications (Table 2-7). Overall, more than 8,000 respirator certifications have been issued since 1972. At the same time, approximately 35 percent of the applications received were denied approval or withdrawn.

The PPT Program maintains the Certified Equipment List on the NIOSH website (NIOSH, 2008j). This searchable database allows employers and other respirator purchasers and users to determine if the respirator-related products they are considering have received NIOSH certification. The Certified Equipment List is also used internationally by countries that require or recommend NIOSH-certified respirators.

Another PPT Program output that is used widely by the user community is the NIOSH Respirator Selection Logic (NIOSH, 2004b), which provides respirator program administrators with a process for respirator selection to protect workers in specific workplaces based on the properties of contaminants, limitations of the equipment, and assigned protection factors. Selection criteria for infectious disease

TABLE 2-7 Number of Respirator Certifications (2001-2007) by Category and Calendar Year

Year	SCBA	Gas Masks	Supplied Air	Particulate	Chemical Cartridge	Particulate Filter	Total per Year
2001	5	3	2	6	58	362	436
2002	25	3	0	4	33	181	246
2003	34	0	1	7	33	114	189
2004	22	2	9	4	16	137	190
2005	6	9	13	8	48	82	166
2006	4	4	5	12	14	99	138
2007	41	10	2	7	20	165	245
Total	137	31	32	48	222	1,140	1,610

NOTE: SCBA = self-contained breathing apparatus.
SOURCE: NIOSH, 2007a, 2008p.

hazards are not included in the respirator selection logic due to the lack of data. Research to correct these deficiencies is continuing.

The outputs resulting from the certified product investigation process include product recalls, product retrofits, and certification rescissions. In FY 2006, 32 investigations were open and a total of 37 were completed (NIOSH, 2007a). User notices are distributed through email and posted on the NIOSH website (previously notices were sent via mass mailings) to inform users of corrective actions that need to be taken to resolve performance problems with NIOSH-certified respirators. Since 2001, 32 user notices have been issued by the PPT Program, the affected respirator manufacturer, the component manufacturer, or a combination of the three. User notices are posted online through the NIOSH website, but there is no requirement that the respirator manufacturer (or distributor) maintain a formal documented listing of employers who have purchased certified equipment. As a result, there is no direct mechanism for employers who purchase respirators to learn about devices that have been recalled or require service, and workers may be put at risk because of this important gap in the process. MSHA has recently recognized this need and has implemented such a program (30 CFR 75.1714-8).

In addition to user notices, the PPT Program also posts concept papers on its website. These concept papers detail certification criteria or other issues under consideration. Stakeholders are asked to provide comments, thereby increasing the transparency of the process and opening opportunities for a wider breadth of expertise to be brought to bear on the issue. Current concept papers include one on powered air-purifying respirator performance criteria (NIOSH, 2008n).

Committee Comments on Relevance to Occupational Safety and Health

The PPT Program's extensive work on respirator certification is highly relevant to occupational safety and health because it provides workers with respirators that have been rigorously tested to meet performance criteria for protection against hazardous respiratory exposures. NIOSH certification is well respected as a thorough assessment of the capabilities of respirator equipment and is the accepted standard in the United States as well as in other countries. The PPT Program continues to work to meet the goal of a 90-day certification process.

The major opportunities to improve the certification process focus on expediting updates to the certification regulations (discussed below), including revisions of outdated certification fee schedules. The committee urges accelerated efforts to significantly revise the fee structure while working to ensure that the current level of funding is retained by the PPT Program and used to expand much-needed research and standards activities (see Chapter 5). Strengthening the product and site audit program is also key.

Federal Regulations and Consensus Standards Setting

Improving respirators, and thereby reducing exposures to respiratory hazards, is in large part an effort focused on updating, refining, and developing the tests and performance criteria that respirators must meet to provide effective protection in the workplace. These effectiveness criteria are implemented through federal regulations and consensus standards. Federal regulations for respirator certification are detailed in 42 CFR Part 84 and aim to assess the efficacy of respirators used in U.S. workplaces as mandated by Occupational Safety and Health Administration (OSHA) workplace regulations. Efforts to change the regulations involve a complex and lengthy federal rule-making process (described below). In addition to federal regulations, criteria for respirator performance are implemented through consensus standards organizations such as the International Organization for Standardization (ISO) and the National Fire Protection Association (NFPA).

Planning and Production Inputs

The PPT Program's efforts in standards and regulations (as applied in this report to the 12 objectives) are focused in NPPTL's Policy and Standard Development Branch. These efforts are informed by ongoing work throughout all aspects of the PPT Program.

The budget for policy and standards development activities in the PPT Program was $1.84 million in FY 2007, the lowest annual total for the years examined by the committee (Table 2-8). Increased funding totals in FY 2002 through

TABLE 2-8 Funding for NIOSH PPT Policy and Standards Development

	FY 2001	FY 2002	FY 2003	FY 2004	FY 2005	FY 2006	FY 2007
Funds expended (million dollars)	2.25	4.34	7.59	4.35	6.69	3.78	1.84

SOURCE: NIOSH, 2007a.

FY 2005 reflect additional resources for the development of CBRN regulations made available through the Department of Homeland Security.

The PPT Program obtains input from manufacturers, employers, employees, and other stakeholders through several venues. This input is used not only in revising federal regulations and consensus standards but also in planning for research priorities, considering changes in certification, and strategic planning. Thus, the following overview of the public input to the PPT Program applies to all PPT Program efforts.

The PPT Program has been active in organizing public meetings (Box 2-1). The work on establishing CBRN respirator standards involved one to two public meetings annually for several years in addition to widespread input from professional organizations and federal agencies. In the early phases of its initiative on total inward leakage (TIL), the PPT Program held a public meeting in July 2004 to gain stakeholder feedback on the concept and testing plan. In addition, input was requested through a *Federal Register* notice. Similarly in June 2007, after completing testing on half-facepiece respirators, the PPT Program held a public meeting to receive further feedback on the TIL efforts. In November 2004, the PPT Program organized the workshop *Respiratory Protection for Infectious Agents* to explore research gaps. The PPT Program's listserv is used to disseminate information to more than 2,500 subscribers.

Peer review panels are another mechanism for receiving input to the PPT Program. In addition to the Institute of Medicine panels described throughout this chapter, the PPT Program has convened peer review teams to assess various parts of its research program. For example, in 2004, a peer review team evaluated the total inward leakage research protocol (NIOSH, 2007a). The PPT Program's work on end-of-service-life (ESLI) indicators for respirator cartridges also benefited from assessment through a formal peer review held in the spring of 2005.

Recently, the PPT Program has begun to solicit the input of the user community through customer surveys. The first survey of manufacturers and users was conducted in 2005. Survey results are posted on the NIOSH website (NIOSH, 2007g). The next survey was in the process of being conducted during the course of this study.

> **BOX 2-1**
> **NIOSH-Sponsored PPT Meetings**
>
> **Public Meetings**
>
> | Date | Major Topic |
> |---|---|
> | March 6, 2008 | PPT Program |
> | March 22, 2007 | LTFE Program Concept |
> | October 12-13, 2006 | New program ideas including total inward leakage |
> | September 28, 2006 | Closed-circuit escape respirators |
> | September 19, 2006 | Closed-circuit escape respirators |
> | April 27, 2006 | Expediting the respirator certification process |
> | December 13, 2005 | CBRN respirator standards |
> | July 19-20, 2005 | CBRN respirator standards |
> | December 15, 2004 | CBRN respirator standards |
> | August 24, 2004 | Total inward leakage requirements |
> | May 4, 2004 | CBRN respirator standards |
> | October 16, 2003 | CBRN respirator standards |
> | June 25, 2003 | CBRN respirator standards |
> | April 29, 2003 | CBRN respirator standards |
> | April 10, 2003 | Standards for respiratory devices |
> | June 18-19, 2002 | CBRN respirator standards |
> | April 4-5, 2001 | Research directions for NPPTL |
>
> **Manufacturer Meetings**
>
> April 10-12, 2007; October 11, 2006; July 21, 2005; April 13, 2005
>
> ---
>
> NOTE: CBRN = chemical, biological, radiological, and nuclear; LTFE = Long-Term Field Evaluation; NPPTL = National Personal Protective Technology Laboratory.

Activities and Outputs

The PPT Program's efforts in policy making and standards setting occur through two major avenues: the federal rule-making process and consensus standards organizations.

Federal regulations Since the certification program is conducted under the auspices of 42 CFR Part 84, it operates with the force of law under the authority of the federal regulatory enforcement statutes and is supported by the federal rule-making process. The federal rule-making process, as outlined in the Administrative Procedure Act (5 USC 5 [511-599]) ensures that the rule is carefully constructed, that the public has full knowledge of the force of the rule, and that there is ample opportunity for those who will be affected by the rule to comment on it in a manner that ensures that the agency will take those comments into account. All of this takes time. Rough estimates are that this is at least a 2- to 3-year process from development of the performance criteria and background documents to enactment of the final rule. The steps in the rule-making process are summarized in Table 2-9.

The PPT Program through NPPTL has developed a modular approach to updating federal regulations. Instead of updating the entire set of respirator certification regulations, the PPT Program is updating sections of the regulations. The overview of the PPT Program's activities and outputs in this area begins with a description of the CBRN standards and then focuses on other regulations that are in the process of being updated.

CBRN respirator certification standards The many-faceted efforts to develop and implement standards for the certification of CBRN respirators have been a

TABLE 2-9 Steps in the Federal Rule-Making Process for Changes to 42 CFR 84

Step		Estimated Time to Completion (months)
1.	Preparation of the proposed rule • Develop conceptual requirements • Finalize technical criteria and standard test procedures • Finalize the preamble	12-24 (these activities take place before the involvement of higher agencies and the OMB)
2.	Conduct higher agency reviews by NIOSH, CDC, and DHHS	6[a]
3.	OMB reviews proposed rule	3
4.	Submit proposed rule for publication in *Federal Register*; open comment period; receive comments regarding the proposed rule in a docket	3
5.	Address comments received in the docket; conduct information exchange public meetings if necessary	3
6.	Prepare final rule and conduct higher agency review	6
7.	OMB review of final rule	3
8.	Publish final rule in *Federal Register*	

NOTE: CDC = Centers for Disease Control and Prevention; DHHS = Department of Health and Human Services; OMB = Office of Management and Budget.
[a]Estimated based on 60 days with each agency.
SOURCE: NIOSH, 2008i.

major focus of the PPT Program since the inception of NPPTL in 2001. After the terrorist attacks on the United States in 2001, efforts were expedited to certify respirators that could provide protection against CBRN threats. As described throughout this report, the CBRN effort involved extensive collaborations with numerous partners and many public meetings. PPT Program staff worked with partner organizations and contractors to collect and evaluate more than 340 standards for respiratory protection equipment from 32 countries and standards organizations (NIOSH, 2007a). Relevant and applicable standards that met the performance requirements were adopted. Further, the toxic industrial chemicals and toxic industrial materials requirements were researched and developed by the PPT Program. A number of public meetings were held to focus on CBRN regulations and obtain stakeholder input. As a part of the efforts to establish CBRN standards for respirators, the PPT Program fast-tracked the development of an exploratory benchmark test to assess the performance of commercially available self-contained breathing apparatus (SCBA) respirators against chemical warfare agents. Existing U.S. Army chemical warfare agent test methods were adapted, and benchmark testing was initially conducted on SCBA respirators that were available to emergency responders in the United States. Testing of CBRN respirators using live agents is conducted by the U.S. Army under an interagency agreement between NIOSH and the U.S. Army Research, Development, and Engineering Command.

Separate CBRN regulatory standards are needed for each of the relevant classes of respirators; part of that process is still under way. The initial regulation, completed in January 2002, was for the certification of SCBA respirators for CBRN exposures; updates to the SCBA regulations were completed in March 2003 (NIOSH, 2008k). Subsequently, the regulations were completed for CBRN gas masks (March 2003), CBRN escape sets (October 2003), and powered air-purifying respirators (PAPRs) (October 2006). The remaining CBRN respirator regulatory standards (for supplied-air respirators, closed-circuit SCBAs, and combination sets) will be completed through the standard (not expedited) rule-making process.

The primary output of these efforts has been the certification of CBRN respirators. From FY 2002 through FY 2007, 45 respirators received CBRN certification and there were 20 certified retrofits (NIOSH, 2008o). The PPT Program has produced a number of guidance documents and fact sheets that are highly relevant to the use of CBRN respirators (e.g., NIOSH, 2004c, 2005c), and PPT Program staff have disseminated information on the CBRN standards through professional conferences (e.g., Boord and Dower, 2002). Additionally, as a result of contracts with Pennsylvania State University and RAND, reports on PPT guidelines for emergency responders were published and distributed (LaTourrette et al., 2003; Ramani et al., 2003).

The PPT Program responded quickly to the challenges of developing and implementing CBRN certification regulations—an effort that involved coordinating with multiple agencies and organizations and was accomplished through a well-organized and open process.

Respirator regulatory changes At the time this report was being prepared, five other modules of the respirator regulations were in various stages of development (Table 2-10). The PPT Program is in the process of developing a draft standard for powered air-purifying respirators that would allow application-specific requirements for PAPRs designed for specific uses, such as hospitals. These respirators are effective against airborne contaminants in an industrial setting, but their high flow rates are impediments to their use in other occupations, such as health care, where the noise level needs to be reduced. The concept paper for the PAPR standard was published on the NIOSH website in January 2008 (NIOSH, 2008n), and the plan is for submission for review in December 2008. Public meetings regarding the updated mine escape respirator (closed-circuit escape SCBA) were held in 2003, the concept paper was published in 2004, and the regulatory revision was submitted for review in July 2007. Regulatory revisions regarding closed-circuit self-breathing apparatus respirators and supplied-air respirators are in development and anticipated to be submitted for review by December 2009. Another of the anticipated regulatory changes focuses on total inward leakage. This regulation will provide improved procedures in the certification process for examining the fit of respirators. Air-purifying respirators have not been required to be evaluated for fit since the revision of 42 CFR Part 84 in 1995. The concept paper regarding total inward leakage was published in 2004 (NIOSH, 2008q), and current plans are to submit it for review in the summer of 2008.

One of the significant sections needing expedited revision is the certification fee schedule. As discussed in the earlier section on the budget for respirator

TABLE 2-10 Status of Federal Regulatory Changes (as of March 2008)

Closed-circuit escape respirator	Submitted for higher agency review in July 2007
Quality assurance module	Submitted for higher agency review in October 2007
Total inward leakage (half-masks and full facepiece respirators)	In development; to be submitted for higher agency review in July-August 2008
Powered air-purifying respirators	In development; to be submitted for higher agency review in December 2008
Closed-circuit self-contained breathing apparatus and supplied-air respirators	In development; to be submitted for higher agency review by December 2009

SOURCE: NIOSH, 2008i.

certification, only a fraction of the costs of respirator certification are borne by the certification fees paid by manufacturers. Because the CBRN regulations have recently been revised, they include the cost of the specialized testing that is done for those respirators, although total costs are still not fully recovered by the PPT Program. Further, product and facility auditing costs are paid with federal funds and should be included as part of the certification fee.

The PPT Program has a goal of completing two regulatory modules per year. This is a reasonable goal and one that the committee believes the PPT Program should be able to meet. The committee sees these revisions and additions to the regulatory standards as a major opportunity for the PPT Program to improve respirator performance through updated tests that address current and evolving technologies (see further discussion below and in Chapter 5).

Consensus standards The PPT Program staff is actively involved in work on developing consensus standards relevant to respirators. Regarding CBRN issues, PPT Program staff work on the relevant NFPA technical committees and assisted in the 2007 revision of NFPA 1981, the *NFPA Standard on Open-Circuit SCBA for Emergency Services*. Work is also ongoing with the ISO Human Factors Committee regarding standards for CBRN respirators.

PPT Program staff members participate on the ASTM committee focused on nanotechnology issues for PPT, as well as on the ISO technical committee that is working on developing standards and guidance documents (NIOSH, 2007a). Similarly, PPT Program staff members are active in efforts to incorporate the results of anthropometric research into ISO consensus standards. The PPT Program is also involved in ongoing efforts with the ASTM technical committee working to develop test methods for biological decontamination procedures for PPT as well as ANSI (American National Standards Institute) Z88 standards for respiratory protection.

Committee Comments on Relevance to Occupational Safety and Health

Federal rule-making and consensus standards are highly relevant to improving the criteria by which respirators are evaluated. Both of these mechanisms offer the opportunity to apply research results directly to product improvement. The federal regulatory work on CBRN standards has been, in many ways, a breakthrough effort by the PPT Program. It has shown the value of a collaborative approach with multiple partnerships, the use of applicable industrial and military technologies, and the value of innovation in expediting the development and publication of new testing and respirator certification standards. The process was open and transparent with significant input from stakeholders. The PPT Program has also been active in a number of highly relevant efforts to improve consensus standards for respirators.

The expedited nature of the changes in CBRN regulations, however, stands in contrast to the lengthy processes for other changes in respirator certification regulations. Most regulations have not been changed significantly in more than 35 years (Federal Register, 1972). For some other regulations the changes have been discussed and in process for five years or more. In 1995, regulations on particulate filters were completed as part of the changes from MSHA regulations (30 CFR Part 11) to public health regulations under the responsibility of NIOSH (42 CFR Part 84). The significant backlog in rule making is delaying the use of new technologies and tools for respirator certification. The PPT Program's recent move toward a modular approach to rule making is a step in the right direction.

Updates to the respirator certification process are constrained by the requirements of federal rule making, which is a time-intensive process. Although a number of external factors play a significant role in the speed of the rule-making process, the committee believes that with increased resources and focused attention, the proposed changes and additions to the regulations could be moved more expeditiously through the rule-making pipeline (see Chapter 5). Many important improvements to respirators are currently being explored by the PPT Program and require the supporting regulatory framework.

An important part of that effort will be accelerating changes to the regulations that set the certification fee structure. As noted above, federal funding is being used to cover more than 90 percent of the costs of the certification process. Because of the robustness of the respirator market, the committee believes that certification costs should be covered by respirator manufacturers, just as PPT manufacturers cover third-party certification costs for other types of PPT. The certification cost is a one-time cost for each type of respirator submitted for testing. After receiving certification, the manufacturer can produce hundreds to millions of that type of product and therefore the certification costs are spread out over many items. The revised fee structure should include all costs of certification, including costs incurred in post-certification auditing. Further, the fee structure needs to incorporate the capacity for an annual adjustment tied to the rising costs of certification based on an audit of certification costs. It is critically important that the federal funds now used to cover certification costs be directed to fund much-needed research for all types of PPT (e.g., protective clothing, respirators, eye protection) across all relevant occupational sectors.

Research

NIOSH has a considerable research portfolio focused on addressing hazardous exposures and respiratory disease. The NIOSH Respiratory Disease Research Program, the topic of another National Academies' review (NRC and IOM, 2008b), addresses the reduction of respiratory disease through the broad hierarchy of occupational health controls (as described in Chapter 1). The focus of the PPT Program's research and of this review is on one aspect of the controls—the personal protective technologies.

The PPT Program's evidence package (NIOSH, 2007a) outlined the following five objectives related to research on reducing exposure to inhalation hazards. Some of these objectives also include components related to the certification process or to federal regulatory or consensus standards.

1. Ensure the availability of mine emergency respirators for escape from mines.
2. Improve reliability and level of protection by developing criteria that influence personal protective equipment designs to better fit the range of facial dimensions of respirator users in the U.S. workforce.
3. Quantify the impacts of various personal protective equipment on viral transmission.
4. Evaluate nanofiber-based fabrics and NIOSH-certified respirators for respiratory protection against nanoparticles.
5. Develop and make available end-of-service-life indicator technologies that reliably sense or model performance to ensure respirator users receive effective respiratory protection.

Planning and Production Inputs

Most of the research conducted through the PPT Program is focused on respiratory-related PPT. In FY 2007, spending for research on protection against respiratory hazards totaled $3.7 million (not including overhead), about 77 percent of the total research budget for the PPT Program or about 28 percent of the PPT Program's total budget (NIOSH, 2007a). As noted above, the PPT Program has held many public meetings, manufacturers' meetings, and conferences to obtain input on its research efforts. This deliberate process of planning and consultation has extended to the development of new capacities for conducting laboratory research. For example, peer reviews and public meetings preceded the decision to establish a fit test and TIL test facility to conduct benchmark testing for respirators. The laboratory has been equipped with aerosol measurement instruments, as well as with equipment that allows PPT Program researchers to examine the impact of respirators on communications and speech transmission.

Activities and Outputs

The PPT Program has conducted a broad array of research efforts that are summarized only briefly in the text below. As with other parts of this report, the analysis is focused on NIOSH's PPT efforts related to protection against inhalation and dermal hazards. Research and other efforts on additional types of PPT (e.g., hearing protection, fall harnesses) are also underway at NIOSH and, as discussed in Chapter 5, should be part of an expanded effort to integrate all PPT work at NIOSH.

Mine escape respirators More than 32,000 coal miners who work underground are required to have access to an employer-supplied self-contained self-rescuer respirator that can be used to escape from a mine fire or other situation resulting in a hazardous atmosphere (NIOSH, 2007a). New requirements from the federal Mine Improvement and New Emergency Response Act of 2006 (MINER Act) include expanded training and improved access to these respirators. The PPT Program works with MSHA on investigations of issues related to SCSRs and participates in investigations of respirators recovered from mine disasters. The PPT Program has identified improvements in mine escape respirators as a priority area and, as mentioned above, has sought public input on design issues. The research portion of the PPT Program's work on mine escape respirators is focused on the development of the next generation of self-contained self-rescuers. Resources for this effort have been limited ($200,000 in FY 2004, $84,483 in FY 2005, and $614,482 in FY 2007; NIOSH, 2008a).

Workshops sponsored by the PPT Program and the National Technology Transfer Center discussed the requirements for the next generation of mine escape respirators and identified a need for dockable and hybrid equipment that combines a lightweight, easy-to-use, self-contained filtering unit with the ability to connect the respirator to additional units of breathable air (without having to remove the respirator). Efforts to develop the performance requirements and certification standards for these new types of respirators are continuing. In 2007, the PPT Program contracted with a private-sector company to design and produce an escape respirator with dockable and hybrid features. A prototype has been developed and is in the testing phase. The PPT Program began a new research project in FY 2008 that is examining the physiologic burden of mine escape devices, but the funding is quite limited.

The PPT Program has also conducted research on training methods and on technologies that may aid in mine escape and has worked with MSHA to develop training modules that were distributed to 1,850 mines in 2006 (NIOSH, 2007a). Surveillance efforts through the long-term field evaluation of SCSRs are an important part of the effort to improve mine safety, and as noted in Chapter 5, the committee urges increased field testing efforts in mines and in other types of work sites that use PPT.

Fit and anthropometrics Research on improving the effectiveness of respirators has focused on the two main areas of concern—the fit and the filter. NIOSH has a long history of research and working with manufacturers and others to improve both the filtration and the fit of a range of respirator types (for example, Coffey et al., 1998a,b). In 2003, the PPT Program began research on the total inward leakage of respirators with the goal of further improving the fit of respirators by quantifying the extent of leakage particularly around the face seal of the respirator. Research by the PPT Program has focused on developing TIL performance characteristics and laboratory tests (NIOSH, 2004a). Extensive testing and research are going into this effort. For example, in 2006, a panel of test subjects participated in tests of 101 models of half-facepiece respirators to assist in refining performance criteria; the results of this study should be published. The proposed criteria for use in the respirator certification process were the topic of a June 2007 public meeting. The PPT Program has recently begun work on studies assessing changes in respirator fit and the effect of weight change on respirator fit.

Another related area of PPT research aims to improve respirator fit by identifying a panel of facial anthropometric characteristics that are representative of the U.S. worker population. Individuals with characteristics that fit the parameters in the panel are recruited to test respirators. The panel characteristics are also used to develop manikin-type head forms for testing. The PPT Program's most recent focus in this area has been on updating the test panel that was developed in the 1970s. The PPT Program developed and implemented (through the work of a contractor) the measurement of approximately 4,000 individuals using traditional measurement tools and/or a three-dimensional scanning system (for a subset of the group) to characterize face and head shapes (Anthrotech, 2004). The results were analyzed by PPT Program researchers and used to develop suggested panels for evaluating half- and full-face respirator fit testing. Publications and presentations on the anthropometric research include work by Zhuang and Bradtmiller (2005) and Zhuang and colleagues (2004, 2005, 2006, 2007). The PPT Program contracted with the Institute of Medicine to examine the anthropometric survey and related research issues, and the resulting Institute of Medicine report (IOM, 2007) provided a number of recommendations for improvements. As a follow-up, the PPT Program developed a detailed response in moving forward in these areas of research (NIOSH, 2008f).

Software developed for the principal component analysis of the anthropometric data is being tested by NIOSH and other partners. The panel developed through the anthropometric research is also being used in work on the total-inward leakage certification requirements, and the head circumference and neck circumference data have been used as part of the new CBRN standard for escape respirators and hoods (NIOSH, 2007a).

New areas of research—pandemic influenza and nanotechnology Recent additions to the intramural research portfolio focus on preparation for pandemic influenza and on nanotechnology.

The growing recognition of the vulnerability of the United States and other countries to the potential for an influenza pandemic and the 2003-2004 outbreaks of severe acute respiratory syndrome (SARS) have focused attention on the availability and use of PPT in the event of a pandemic, particularly for healthcare workers involved in the front line of defense against infectious disease. The PPT Program's research on pandemic influenza began in FY 2006. PPT Program researchers are conducting projects focused on the efficacy of decontamination methods for filtering facepiece respirators, the duration of the viability of the influenza virus on PPT, and the effectiveness of respirators or respirator-surgical mask combinations (NIOSH, 2007a). Other research efforts are focused on examining biocidal technologies and their use in respirators. Research being conducted in collaboration with West Virginia University is focused on understanding the production of aerosols by human coughs. The focus of recent research has been guided in part by the issues identified by two IOM reports (IOM, 2006, 2008). The PPT Program contracted with the IOM for a study specifically on the PPT needs of healthcare workers in the event of pandemic influenza (IOM, 2008). Recently the PPT Program released its response to the report and its action plan for following up on the report's recommendations (NIOSH, 2008g).

The resources devoted by the PPT Program to pandemic influenza research have declined from an initial budget of nearly $1.5 million in FY 2006 to approximately $780,000 in FY 2007 and $480,000 in FY 2008 (Table 2-2). Despite the importance of the research on PPT for pandemic influenza hazards and its relevance to protecting workers, there is concern that the priority may be shifting away from this issue even though much important work remains undone. Although there is evidence that the PPT Program has leveraged its minimal resources effectively in this area by sponsoring conferences and reports that have served to identify critical issues, the resources for a comprehensive research program to deal with those issues are lacking.

The PPT Program's outputs regarding pandemic influenza preparedness include interagency efforts and workshops (see above), in addition to publications (Roberge, 2008a,b) and presentations (e.g., Gardner et al., 2006). The 2004 workshop *Respiratory Protection for Infectious Agents* was organized by the PPT Program to identify research gaps. Information from this workshop has been incorporated into NIOSH research proposals (NIOSH, 2007a).

The PPT Program began its work in nanotechnology in FY 2005 by examining the efficiency of NIOSH-approved respirator filter materials in protecting against aerosol particles of 20 to 100 nm. The PPT Program has also funded research in a collaborative effort with the Center for Filtration Research at the University of Minnesota to examine the filtration of nanoparticles between 3 and 20 nm (Kim et al., 2007). The PPT Program is part of the efforts of the NIOSH-wide Nanotechnology Research Center, and PPT Program staff members have participated with other NIOSH colleagues in developing the NIOSH strategic plan on nanotechnology (NIOSH, 2005a). The PPT Program is also involved in research on the use of nanotechnology as applied to PPT. In particular, PPT Program staff conducted a set of studies on the use of respirator filter media that incorporated nanofiber materials. The studies were appropriately terminated due to challenges in developing adequate samples.

The investment in nanotechnology-related research has averaged approximately $315,000 annually from FY 2006 to FY 2008 (Table 2-2), and the committee believes that the PPT Program has made appropriately focused decisions given its limited resources. The more important issue of respirator face seal leakage is in the early phases of research. Leakage is an important question since it is known that leakage around the face seal is the weakest part of a negative-pressure respirator, and nanoparticles are more likely to penetrate leaks than are larger particles. Manikin-based tests are likely to raise more questions than answers. Therefore, fieldwork will likely be necessary to determine the impact of ultrafine particles on leakage and exposure and the impact of this program on worker health. The PPT Program evidence package also indicated that research is being considered regarding the role of nanotechnology-based sensors, which may hold promise for future PPT efforts.

Although, its work on nanotechnology is in its early phases, contributions have been made by the PPT Program including input into the NIOSH strategic plan on nanotechnology (NIOSH, 2005a) and a focused look by NIOSH at nanotechnology issues in the workplace, *Approaches to Safe Nanotechnology* (NIOSH, 2007d). PPT Program staff members have made a number of conference presentations in this area, and the PPT Program has been involved in peer-reviewed publications on respirators and nanoparticles (Kim et al., 2007; Rengasamy et al., 2007).

End-of-service-life indicators An ongoing issue in respirator use has been identifying accurate methods of determining the end of the service life of the carbon-based materials used in air-purifying respirators. OSHA regulations (29 CFR 1910.134) mandate that employers use a formal change schedule or an end-of-service-life indicator. The PPT Program's research in this area began with a focus on the development of software models to provide users with a method for predicting the cartridge service life. The *Breakthrough* software was released in 2004 (NIOSH, 2005b). The newer *MultiVapor* software, designed to assess breakthrough times and service lives for air-purifying respirator cartridges for multiple organic vapors, was released in May 2007 (NIOSH, 2007e). Both are available on CD-ROM; the *MultiVapor* software is also available on the OSHA website with more than 4,500 downloads (NIOSH, 2007a,e); several published peer-reviewed journal articles have provided more detailed information (Wood, 2004, 2005). Recent work by the PPT Program, in collaboration with Carnegie Mellon University, several manufacturers, and others, focuses on sensor systems to detect gases and vapors and provide a signal indicating breakthrough (see Chapter 3). The second phase of the ESLI research program focuses on the development of a sensor that can be embedded in the cartridge and detect vapor breakthrough (King et al., 2007; see further details below and in Chapter 3).

Committee Comments on Relevance to Occupational Safety and Health

The PPT Program's research relevant to respiratory exposures encompasses a wide range of efforts to improve respirators and respirator-related technologies. The PPT Program has moved the research agenda forward in many important directions and has become involved in a number of cutting-edge issues and technologies. The PPT Program has sponsored timely conferences and developed relevant research initiatives regarding respiratory protection in an influenza pandemic. However, many research questions remain, and additional resources would allow the PPT Program to develop wide-ranging partnerships with industry and academia to address additional high-priority areas of research.

The committee believes that NIOSH has made important strides in forwarding the knowledge base on facial anthropometrics and on respirator fit and total inward leakage. The significance of a user seal check to determine or confirm individual respirator fit requires additional investigation by the PPT Program. At the same time, the committee urges a strong and sustained focus on exploring materials sciences and other technologies that may obviate the need for fit testing and improve the individualized fit of PPT. Given the challenges in the workplace of fit testing workers and ensuring that they have proper equipment, the greatest need is for simplifying or eliminating the fitting process. The PPT Program is sponsoring an upcoming workshop to explore new technologies that could provide "fits-all" or "universal-fit" respirators that could easily and effectively conform to fit all face types; further efforts on this topic are needed.

The PPT Program has provided extensive outreach opportunities for input from the general public, manufacturers, employers, and state and federal agencies. The PPT Program is also engaged in a number of partnerships that are effective in leveraging available resources. More should be done to further training efforts on PPT use and to provide data to employers and employees on the effectiveness of PPT in the workplace.

GOALS 2 AND 3: REDUCE EXPOSURES TO DERMAL AND INJURY HAZARDS

In addition to respiratory hazards, many U.S. workers face daily exposures to hazardous chemicals or other toxicants that could potentially be absorbed through the skin; other workers deal with the potential for injury from heat, falls, noise, heavy or sharp objects, and a range of other hazards. NIOSH is currently working through several of its divisions to address relevant PPT aimed at mitigating these occupational hazards. NIOSH's efforts that are reviewed in this report focus on the 12 objectives the committee was asked to examine, of which 4 objectives are related to dermal and injury hazards.

The PPT Program's work on reducing exposures to dermal and injury hazards is accomplished through research and participation in standards-setting efforts. The PPT Program does not have certification responsibilities for protective clothing, gloves, or any other type of dermal or injury PPT. Some of those products are certified by third-party organizations (e.g., Safety Equipment Institute, Underwriters Laboratory) or are manufactured to meet specific consensus standards.

The relevant dermal and injury objectives for this review as identified by the PPT Program follow:

- Improve chemical-barrier protective clothing testing and use practices to reduce worker exposure to chemical dermal hazards.
- Improve emergency responder protective clothing to reduce exposure to thermal, biological, and chemical dermal hazards.
- Investigate physiological and ergonomic impact of protective ensembles on individual wearers in affecting worker exposure to dermal hazards.
- Develop and evaluate warning devices for fire services.

In contrast to exposures to hazards via the respiratory route, which usually have well-characterized guidelines and standards for safe occupational exposure levels, dermal hazards and safe occupational exposure levels are poorly defined. Thus, the primary challenges for dermal PPT are to understand the level of protection needed for different sectors (i.e., industrial, pharmaceutical, healthcare, and agricultural workers) and then utilize the tactical approaches identified above to systematically address the health and safety of workers in these various sectors. In addition to evaluating the protection offered by protective clothing and gloves, a wearer's ability to carry out his or her job efficiently and effectively while wearing the PPT must be addressed. Thus, issues regarding dermal PPT include dermal hazard assessment, permeation of hazards through the skin and through protective clothing or other PPT, physiological and ergonomic impact of the PPT, durability, and decontamination and reuse.

Planning and Production Inputs

Only a small percentage (10 percent in FY 2007) of the PPT Program's total budget is allocated for dermal and injury-related efforts (Table 2-2). In large part this is due to NIOSH's historical focus and congressional mandate on respirator certification and on improving the quality and effectiveness of respirators. In FY 2007, $1,142,320 was designated in the PPT Program's budget for work on reducing hazardous dermal exposures and $176,453 for work on the one objective related to reducing exposure to injury hazards (data include overhead costs; Table 2-2). Other efforts at NIOSH are focused on PPT for injury prevention but are not included in these budget figures. Similarly, only a small number of staff members are involved in work on reducing dermal exposures. In FY 2008, out of a total of slightly more than 70 total FTEs in the PPT Program, 4.6 worked on projects related to dermal exposures, and the staff allocation for work on the sensor system for reduction of injury hazards was 0.6 FTE (Table 2-3). The laboratory facilities for the PPT Program's intramural dermal research program have expanded in recent years with the addition of the aerosol laboratory and human research physiology laboratory in 2005. The committee regards this as a step in the right direction.

The committee compiled a rough timeline specific to the PPT Program's inputs, activities, and outputs related to dermal exposures (Box 2-2). Of note in the planning inputs is the 1998 NORA (National Occupational Research Agenda) conference *Setting the Research Agenda for Control of Workplace Hazards for the 21st Century*, which identified some of NIOSH's research priorities in this area.

The PPT Program has heightened the relevance of its work in dermal and injury PPT by seeking input from workers, manufacturers, professional associations, employers, and many others through a variety of different venues. At a Centers for Disease Control and Prevention (CDC) stakeholders meeting in April 2001, 16 emergency responders met and developed a 5-year concept research plan relevant to protective clothing (CDC, 2001). As part of its response to the terrorist events of September 2001, the PPT Program organized a conference in December 2001 to hear from emergency responders, firefighters, and others on what needed to be done to improve PPT for responding to such events. As noted above in the discussion on respirator-related standards, the PPT Program holds frequent public meetings and provides multiple avenues for stakeholder input. Most of the public meetings have focused on respirator-related issues, but recent meetings, particularly the March 2008 public meeting, have had a broader focus that included multiple types of PPT.

> **BOX 2-2**
> **Timeline of Key Events for the Dermal PPT Program—Inputs, Activities, and Outputs**
>
> *1998*
> - NORA workshop, *Setting the Research Agenda*
>
> *2001*
> - CDC-sponsored emergency responder stakeholder meeting
> - Research studies initiated on decontamination methods
> - Conference focusing on PPT for emergency workers
>
> *2003*
> - Protective clothing lab established at NPPTL
>
> *2004*
> - MOU established between NIOSH and TSWG to evaluate next-generation structural firefighting PPT with chemical or biological protection
>
> *2005*
> - Intramural research begun on Project HEROES®
> - MOUs established between NIOSH and ASTM and between NIOSH and NFPA
> - Decontamination work used to develop AIHA guideline
> - Aerosol laboratory and physiology laboratory established
> - Conference on protecting first responders
> - EMS protective clothing project begun
>
> *2007*
> - Permeation calculator released
> - MOU established between TSWG and NIOSH to collaborate on permeation criteria initiatives
>
> NOTE: AIHA = American Industrial Hygiene Association; EMS = Emergency Medical Services; HEROES = Homeland Emergency Response Operational and Equipment Systems; MOU = memorandum of understanding; TSWG = Technical Support Working Group.

Activities and Outputs

Intramural research on dermal protection began in NIOSH before the PPT Program was established; several of the projects were transferred in 2001 when NPPTL was created. Other projects, particularly on dermal hazard assessment, remain in the NIOSH divisions working in those areas.

A series of intramural NIOSH studies in the late 1990s and early 2000s (transferred to NPPTL after 2001) focused on the development of colorimetric or sorbent indicators for assessing chemical permeation through gloves. NIOSH researchers worked on indicators that could be incorporated into the inside of gloves so that they would change color when exposed to specific hazardous chemicals (i.e., after permeation through the glove). After a number of NIOSH studies and publications (e.g., Vo, 2004), further work in this area was deemed to be most appropriate for the private sector.

Permeation and Decontamination

Decontamination of chemical protective clothing was identified as a priority research area in the 1998 workshop *Control of Workplace Hazards* (NIOSH, 2007a), with goals of developing suitable methods and procedures for effectively decontaminating and extending the useful life of chemical protective clothing. The PPT Program's research has involved intramural tests on the degradation of materials in chemical protective clothing as a result of decontamination processes and the effectiveness of a variety of decontamination approaches. The PPT Program has contracted with a private-sector lab to conduct permeation testing and also has had a contract with the University of California, Davis, to explore the concept of developing self-decontaminating functional textiles and polymers for protective clothing. This research has contributed to the knowledge base on decontamination and reuse. However, much remains to be learned on efficient and effective decontamination methods. PPT Program staff members have been active in working with the American Industrial Hygiene Association (AIHA) in the development of the AIHA guideline on the decontamination of chemical protective clothing and equipment (see Chapter 3).

The PPT Program's research on dermal protection has resulted in the development of a permeation calculator that utilizes the results of chemical protective clothing permeation experiments (e.g., using ASTM test methods) to derive parameters such as steady-state permeation rate and breakthrough detection time (Gao et al., 2005; NIOSH, 2008b). The permeation calculator is available on the NIOSH website or on CD.

More recently, the PPT Program is exploring decontamination issues relevant to protective clothing used by emergency responders to better understand how the wear-and-tear that these products undergo on a daily basis impacts cleaning and decontamination. Work on this project is being done in concert with a private-sector firm and through interactions with NFPA and ASTM International technical committees.

One of the critical needs for improving protective clothing relates to the determination of parameters that may better reflect actual skin exposure as a result of permeation through the protective clothing. To this end, efforts are focused on assessing cumulative permeation of chemical warfare agents and toxic industrial chemicals and linking the results of these assessments to the development of dermal exposure limits for those chemicals. A recent memorandum of understanding (MOU) between NIOSH and the Technical Support Working Group (TSWG) of the Department of Defense establishes collaborative efforts focused on understanding and defining risk-based permeation criteria. The InterAgency Board for Equipment Standardization and Interoperability (IAB) identified this topic as a priority for first responders. The PPT Program's role in this partnership includes providing input in the development of the permeation model, development and review of the skin permeation test plan, and the review of model predictions (NIOSH, 2007h). Other partners in the effort to develop permeation criteria include NFPA, ASTM International, the Canadian Royal Military College, and two private-sector companies. The development of standards and testing methods for a wider array of chemicals is needed and would offer a significant contribution to the goal of utilizing quantitative risk assessment as input to developing and selecting appropriate chemical protective clothing.

Relevant to the work on cumulative permeation for dermal risk assessment are the skin notation efforts under way in other divisions at NIOSH. While the work of the PPT Program will help determine the exposure variable of the risk equation, information on the hazard variable is also seriously lacking. To perform adequate quantitative risk assessments both exposure and hazard data are needed. The committee hopes that the skin notation work can be expanded to include more quantifiable characterization of dermal hazards.

New initiatives are focused on examining the penetration of nanoparticles through protective clothing and on developing new approaches for measuring aerosol particle penetration through protective clothing. The PPT Program is working with the Nanotech Consortium on this effort, and partners include private- and public-sector agencies and organizations.

Emergency Response—PPT Needs and Physiologic Burden

The PPT Program contracted with the International Association of Fire Fighters for a report that provided a detailed description of the PPT needs of firefighters and provided recommendations on research priorities for moving forward in addressing these evolving needs (IAFF, 2003). This report was used by the PPT Program and extramural researchers in developing research priorities and planning research initiatives. Another report focused on reviewing gaps and limitations in test methods for firefighters and emergency responders (Barker, 2005). This report provided a basis for the PPT Program and extramural efforts to develop new test methods, including a test to evaluate stored energy effects in materials used in the construction of firefighter suits, and protocols for assessing physiological issues associated with the performance of protective ensembles. The challenge with limited resources is to transfer these technologies and advances from firefighting to other work sectors (e.g., agricultural workers, welders, abrasive blasting).

Physiological effects related to ergonomic factors are widely recognized as highly relevant in determining the performance of PPT used by emergency responders. Research on the physiologic burdens of protective clothing has been a focus of research in the PPT Program, particularly related to firefighter ensembles and the work of the International Association of Fire Fighters' collaborative effort Project HEROES® (Homeland Emergency Response Operational and Equipment Systems), in conjunction with TSWG, the Department of Homeland Security, the International Association of Fire Chiefs, the University of Massachusetts, the University of Arkansas, and a private-sector manufacturing company. The PPT Program's research and testing efforts related to this project focus on assessing the physiologic burdens of firefighter ensembles. In 2005, the physiology laboratory was established by the PPT Program. The lab is used for this project as well as other measures of the physiologic burden of PPT. Recent research has focused on testing a number of cooling devices incorporated in protective clothing. Additional focus on the ergonomic aspects of protective clothing ensembles is key to future efforts.

Research, conducted through collaboration with North Carolina State University, has focused on the firefighter protective ensemble and the impact of stored thermal energy. This research is developing testing protocols designed to evaluate the effects of firefighter turn-out materials on skin burn injuries associated with exposure to certain thermal environments in structural firefighting operations. This research is relevant to addressing that hazard in the firefighting community. Results of the project will be used to implement this laboratory testing method in the NFPA 1971 *Standard on Protective Ensembles for Structural Fire Fighting and Proximity Fire Fighting*. The knowledge base is limited regarding the physiological burdens of PPT relevant to industry sectors beyond emergency responders; further efforts are needed to improve the PPT needs of other work sectors including agricultural and construction workers.

Warning Devices

As a part of its role in the NIOSH Fire Fighter Fatality Investigation and Prevention Program, the PPT Program has been involved in examining personal alert safety system (PASS) equipment. PASS devices are important safety equipment for firefighters, sounding an audible alarm when firefighters are motionless or when activated by firefighters in trouble. This audible alarm helps other firefighters locate those in trouble.

In 2005, NIOSH notified NFPA of several fatal firefighter incidents investigated by NIOSH in which the PASS device would have been expected to function, but was not heard or was barely audible. Reasons the PASS device may not have performed as designed were examined by NIOSH and by NIST. PPT Program staff participated in the NFPA Technical Committee on Electronic Safety Equipment to revise the relevant standards. The PPT Program continues to be involved, although with limited resources, in efforts to improve and enhance the reliability of PASS devices. Since NIOSH does not certify these devices it does not have the authority to recall older models of the device. New performance requirements in the revised NFPA standard only address the equipment certified to the new standard. Devices similar to PASS should be evaluated for use by the increasing number of workers who work alone, in confined spaces, or with limited communication options.

Collaborations

As evidenced by all of the above, the PPT Program works with numerous private- and public-sector partners to carry out its work on dermal PPT. Efforts to establish MOUs are activities that require time and resources and yield multiple benefits through the partnerships established. NIOSH has established a memorandum of understanding with ASTM and with NFPA and has several MOUs with the Technical Support Working Group including one to evaluate structural firefighting PPT with chemical or biological protection. In addition to partnerships with other agencies and organizations, another major way in which the PPT Program has made the most of its limited resources is through participation in consensus standards development efforts. PPT Program staff actively participate in ASTM, AIHA, and NFPA committees, and as described in Chapter 3, much of this participation has resulted in the development and refinement of consensus standards that improve the testing and certification of PPT. PPT Program staff have also been active in the work of the IAB, an organization focused on the equipment needs of first responders with an emphasis on chemical, biological, radiological, nuclear, or explosive issues. PPT Program staff members have served in leadership roles in the Interagency Board's Federal Coordinating Committee and Personal Protective and Operational Equipment Subgroup.

In 2005, the PPT Program, in collaboration with the Department of Industrial and Systems Engineering at Virginia Tech, sponsored the conference *Advanced Personal Protective Equipment: Challenges in Protecting First Responders*, which brought together more than 150 emergency responders to learn about new initiatives and to share ideas on next steps for PPT in this field (Virginia Tech, 2005).

Committee Comments on Relevance to Occupational Safety and Health

The PPT Program has effectively leveraged it minimal resources in the area of reducing exposure to dermal hazards, in terms of both planning and implementation. By employing various worker and stakeholder forums to obtain input on the needs of the fire service and emergency responder communities, the PPT Program has refined the research agenda to focus on issues relevant to these worker communities. Further, the PPT Program has not only utilized its own intramural laboratory but also worked collaboratively with others in industry, academia, and professional associations to move forward in improving dermal PPT, particularly for the firefighter and emergency response communities. The PPT Program has developed a wide range of partnerships but might benefit from collaborations or consultations with the Human Factors and Ergonomics Society as well as others with expertise in human factors issues.

The committee finds the PPT Program's work on physiological challenges, ensemble testing, decontamination, and chemical permeation testing to be relevant to making progress in improving dermal protection. Research projects undertaken during the initial years of the PPT Program were fairly limited in scope and approach, but recent efforts have made substantive progress in partnering with other agencies and organizations to conduct research that is more focused on improving worker safety and health.

The risk assessment work based on cumulative permeation is a good start in a high-priority area. If this work is expanded to a wide variety of chemicals, and particularly if it is coupled with dermal permeation work performed in other NIOSH divisions, it will make a significant contribution toward improving chemical protective clothing. Because of limited information on the actual hazard that many chemicals pose to the skin and the lack of developed and standardized methods for assessing actual skin exposure, both with and without the use of chemical protective clothing, most selection decisions have one of two outcomes: select the best chemical protective clothing based solely or mostly on permeation performance, or select the cheapest products that will not degrade when exposed. The former tends to ignore other selection factors such as dexterity, tactility, and puncture resistance. The latter ignores the fact that although degradation of chemical protective clothing may not occur in use, permeation may lead to unacceptable skin exposures. Thus, better risk assessment data are needed both to improve the rationale for the selection of chemical protective clothing and to confirm that chosen products are indeed providing the anticipated protection.

To determine the effectiveness of chemical protective clothing, field performance evaluations are needed and should be expanded. Although laboratory permeation tests are relative indicators of protection, in actual field use many other factors may modify the effectiveness of these products. Such factors include the construction of the protective clothing, temperature, exposures to chemical mixtures, decontamination, and cleaning. The only way to be sure that chemical protective clothing is working is to evaluate it in the field. Thus, techniques that are standardized, valid, reliable, and relatively easy to apply are needed.

The PPT Program is helping to lead efforts to address the critical areas of ensemble testing and physiological effects of PPT. One of the challenges in developing PPT is to address relevant gender and anthropometric differences that may affect the fit, wear, and use of the equipment. A recent PPT Program research study evaluated the physiological impact of the weight of firefighter footwear and included female test subjects. As the research on dermal PPT moves beyond efficacy and toward effectiveness, it will be critical to address a broad range of human factors (Chapter 4).

Much of the work in dermal PPT has revolved around PPT for emergency responders, with only minimal work done to address the needs of workers in other sectors. In large part, this has been the result of the PPT Program's making best use of limited resources and connecting with partners in the emergency response community that have a heightened interest in PPT issues. However, the committee recognizes that PPT needs vary widely among occupations—the needs of a pesticide applicator are quite different from those of a firefighter, as are the PPT needs of a nurse or of a pharmaceutical manufacturing worker. The committee urges wider efforts targeted at dermal PPT, with increased resources enabling the PPT Program to address the needs of a wide range of occupations across the broad spectrum of PPT.

SURVEILLANCE

A cornerstone program of PPT research, certification, and standards should be an active program of surveillance that produces information on occupational hazards and exposures, employer practices, and the use of PPT in the workplace. This strategy would be consistent with the overall emphasis that NIOSH places on surveillance as a foundation for its programs.

Since its creation by the Occupational Safety and Health Act of 1970, NIOSH has emphasized a program of surveillance to track occupational injuries, illnesses, and hazards. Surveillance activities have often documented U.S. progress in reducing the burden of work-related diseases and injuries, and have served to identify problems that require additional research and prevention efforts. Such efforts are likely to translate into successful interventions in the workplace. However, relatively little attention has been paid to understanding the interaction between the particular exposures, hazards, and practices in the workplace that are relevant to optimizing personal protective technology. In the 1970s and 1980s, NIOSH sponsored a national hazard survey and database. Then, in the late 1990s, the agency again considered options for producing information on hazards and exposures. The study of options by a multidisciplinary team of NIOSH staff representing various NIOSH organizations (the Respirator Surveillance Team) led to a decision to sponsor a national survey of respirator use in the workplace (Campbell et al., 1998). Thus, planning for the survey that would be conducted by the Bureau of Labor Statistics for NIOSH was well under way when NPPTL was founded.

Planning and Production Inputs

On an ongoing basis, the surveillance component is a small part of the PPT Program, accounting for about 3 percent of the overall PPT budget in FY 2007 and about the same in FY 2008. These funds support a small program that focuses on analysis and dissemination of the 7-year-old findings of the national survey of respirator use in the workforce, developing an action plan to address the recommendations of a report provided by the National Academies (NRC, 2007), and respirator interventions at construction work sites in collaboration with industry groups.

Activities and Outputs

NIOSH surveillance and tracking data for the PPT Program have been funneled largely through one data source: the Bureau of Labor Statistics (BLS)-NIOSH 2001 nationwide respirator survey, *Survey of Respirator Use and Practices* (SRUP). The purpose of the survey was to help NIOSH better understand respirator and other PPT use and practices, with the ultimate goal of using interventions to improve respirator programs. The target population for the survey was private-sector respirator users with unemployment insurance programs who were included in the 1999 Survey of Occupational Injuries and Illnesses. The results of the survey were used to identify industries that have a high rate of respiratory protection use. The survey results also led to the conclusion that until adequate engineering controls are available and widely implemented, it is likely that respirators will continue to be used—especially in the construction sector. A survey report entitled *Respirator Usage in Private Sector Firms* (BLS and NIOSH, 2003) described the findings of the NIOSH-BLS survey.

In 2007, PPT researchers continued to mine the findings of this survey, publishing numerous articles and making presentations at professional conferences to disseminate results across a number of different industries, including agriculture, forestry and fishing, manufacturing, construction, transportation, demolition, and mining (NIOSH, 2007a). Findings were also specifically described with respect to existing employer programs and other aspects of optimizing respirator fit among workers. Overall, the survey report and subsequent publications and presentations provide a limited description of the state of respirator use and corresponding programs in the workplace, as well as recommendations for future improvement.

In the years since the SRUP survey, PPT Program researchers have also focused on developing a research protocol and follow-up research study as a next step toward gathering additional PPE surveillance data. Follow-up activities involved conducting focus groups and other work with the construction industry to identify intervention strategies. The PPT Program has concentrated on collaboration with industry groups to develop successful respirator program concepts that could be considered for application in the construction sector. Recently the PPT Program developed an action plan and framework for future surveillance work in conjunction with other divisions at NIOSH (NIOSH, 2008h). Proposed efforts include building on existing surveys and potentially conducting a pilot study focused on PPT use in the healthcare and social assistance work sector.

The efforts of the PPT Program to expand surveillance in order to better understand the interplay between hazards, exposure, and respirator use in the workplace are under the auspices of, and must be generally consistent with, the surveillance objectives of NIOSH. These objectives are outlined in the NIOSH Surveillance Strategic Plan (NIOSH, 2001), which calls for better coordination of surveillance activities between all federal and state agencies responsible for worker protection. The strategic plan also calls for a series of NIOSH-wide initiatives, such as the development of a comprehensive, nationally representative exposure survey and a national occupational exposure surveillance database. The plan affords the possibility of leveraging the surveillance initiatives of NIOSH to inform the development of improved protective equipment.

Committee Comments on Relevance to Occupational Safety and Health

The committee believes that surveillance and dissemination efforts within the PPT Program have a high level of relevance. Further, the committee concludes that the results of the 2001 survey of respirator use in industry, while subject to some limitations outlined in a previous NRC report (NRC, 2007), nonetheless could serve as a prototype for going forward as NIOSH structures the dissemination of new information about respirator use across industries and users.

OVERALL ASSESSMENT OF RELEVANCE

In considering the relevance of the PPT Program's efforts, the committee examined 12 of the program's objectives across the three principal domains of research, respirator certification, and policy and standards setting. The committee took into account the major external factors, particularly the limited budget and the regulatory mandate for respirator certification. The PPT Program operates in a set of multiple, small, partly refurbished laboratories dispersed over several acres. These facilities are inadequate for the challenges of overseeing the development of state-of-the-art PPT that must protect the health and safety of the nation's workers.

The respirator certification program is a premier function of the PPT Program. Since 2001, more than 1,600 respirators have been certified, and substantive progress is being made in meeting the congressional mandate of completing certification within 90 days. However, having a long-standing spotlight on respirators, compounded by budget limitations, constrains efforts to address other types of PPT (e.g., protective clothing, eye protection). Recent efforts, particularly in consensus standards setting, seem to be appropriately broadening the scope of the PPT Program.

NIOSH is one of only a few federal agencies that has on-site certification testing responsibilities and facilities. Because OSHA and MSHA require employers to purchase only NIOSH-certified respirators, NIOSH certification is viewed by manufacturers and employers as a business necessity. NIOSH certification regulations are in use by other countries as a model or basis for their respirator certification efforts. The PPT Program conducts a limited number of product audits and conducts manufacturer site audits using both staff and external consultants. Efforts to ensure the effectiveness of respirators would be strengthened through increased resources that could be directed toward field testing and expedited revision of the federal certification regulations.

The PPT Program has had well-documented success in its quick turnaround in developing the CBRN federal respirator standards. This effort involved extensive collaborative efforts with other federal agencies, nonprofit organizations, manufacturers, and others. The PPT Program is in the midst of updating the regulations regarding the certification of mine self-rescue respirators. The PPT Program has conducted relevant research on total inward leakage, which is a major concern in respiratory protection, and on issues focused on criteria for powered air-purifying respirator regulations. However, the regulatory standards related to these issues are still in the initial stages of the rule-making process and expedited efforts are needed to move the process forward.

Consensus standards-setting activities are another priority area for the PPT Program and one in which staff members have been active in the technical committees that are highly relevant to the program's work. Participation in the development of ASTM, ANSI, NFPA, and ISO standards and test methods has been the primary mechanism for the PPT Program's productive engagement in standards designed to reduce hazardous dermal exposures. PPT Program research has also contributed to test methods and performance standards for protective gear.

The PPT Program is proactive in obtaining input from a range of stakeholders through a series of public meetings and manufacturers' meetings focused on specific topics or proposed changes to the certification regulations. Website and listserv capabilities are utilized for dissemination of invitations to upcoming public meetings, user notices, the Certified Equipment List, guidelines, and other key information. In the last few years, the PPT Program has become active in collaborations with various federal agencies and other partners and has begun to explore links with extramural researchers. As discussed in its recommendations (Chapter 5), the committee urges a concentrated effort to bring the breadth of expertise in the extramural research community to bear on intramural and other pertinent PPT research questions.

The time frame for the committee's review began with the inception of NPPTL in 2001. In this relatively short period of time, the program has initiated a range of relevant research projects. Some of the projects are the result of opportunities driven by external factors and funding, whereas others have been initiated by PPT Program investigators. Recent research initiatives have focused on PPT for pandemic influenza and others have focused on efforts to examine the as-yet largely unknown implications of exposure to the products and by-products of nanotechnology. In addition to research to support and improve the respirator certification program (e.g., total inward leakage, anthropometrics), the committee suggests that the PPT Program address research in priority areas, particularly those for mining emergencies, dermal protection, and heat-related hazards. Limitations in the research budget are a major impediment to further improvements in PPT ensembles and in work that is needed across a range of occupations (e.g., agriculture, industry, construction, health care). While research has focused largely on engineering aspects of PPT, one of the challenges to be addressed in the near future is improving and ensuring usability. This will require particular emphasis on increasing safety by improving the comfort, wearability, and individual and organizational incentives needed to ensure that workers do in fact wear PPT.

On the basis of its review of the PPT Program's work in research, certification, and policy and standards setting, the committee has assigned the NIOSH Personal Protective Technology Program a score of 4 for relevance. This score reflects the judgment that the PPT Program is working in priority areas and is engaged in

> **BOX 2-3**
> **Scoring Criteria for Relevance**
>
> 5 = The program's work is in high-priority subject areas, and NIOSH is significantly engaged in appropriate transfer activities for completed projects or reported results.
> 4 = The program's work is in priority subject areas, and NIOSH is engaged in appropriate transfer activities for completed projects or reported results.
> 3 = The program's work is in high-priority or priority subject areas, but NIOSH is not engaged in appropriate transfer activities; or the focus is on lesser priorities, but NIOSH is engaged in appropriate transfer activities.
> 2 = The program is focused on lesser priorities, and NIOSH is not engaged in or planning some appropriate transfer activities.
> 1 = The program is not focused on priorities, and NIOSH is not engaged in transfer activities.

transferring its research into improved products and processes (see Box 2-3 and Appendix A). In the judgment of the committee, the program, with additional resources and an expanded focus, could further improve its relevance score by strengthening the product and site audit programs; expediting revisions to the federal regulatory standards; better harnessing the capabilities of the extramural research community; and placing a stronger emphasis on comfort, wearability, and other human factors that affect workers' use of PPT.

REFERENCES

Anthrotech. 2004. *A head-and-face anthropometric survey of U.S. respirator users: Final report.* Prepared by B. Bradtmiller and M. Friess for NIOSH/NPPTL.

Barker, R. 2005. *A review of gaps and limitations in test methods for first responder protective clothing.* http://www.cdc.gov/niosh/npptl/pdfs/ProtClothEquipReview.pdf (accessed January 22, 2008).

BLS (Bureau of Labor Statistics) and NIOSH (National Institute for Occupational Safety and Health). 2003. *Respirator usage in private sector firms, 2001.* http://www.cdc.gov/niosh/docs/respsurv/ (accessed January 22, 2008).

Boord, L., and J. Dower. 2002. *NIOSH CBRN respiratory protection standards update.* International Society for Respiratory Protection, September 29-October 3, Edinburgh, Scotland.

Campbell, D., A. Dieffenbach, D. Groce, R. A. Jajosky, and G. Spransy. 1998. *Surveillance team report to DRDS lead team.* NIOSH. September 15.

CDC (Centers for Disease Control and Prevention). 2001. *2nd National Stakeholders' Meeting Report, April 10-11.* http://www.cdc.gov/nedss/Archive/Stakeholder2/stakeholder_mtg_2.htm (accessed April 9, 2008).

Coffey, C. C., D. L. Campbell, W. R. Myers, Z. Zhuang, and S. Das. 1998a. Comparison of six respirator fit test methods with an actual measurement of exposure in a simulated health-care environment: Part I—Protocol development. *American Industrial Hygiene Association Journal* 59:852-861.

Coffey, C. C., D. L. Campbell, W. R. Myers, Z. Zhuang, and S. Das. 1998b. Comparison of six respirator fit test methods with an actual measurement of exposure in a simulated health-care environment: Part II—Method comparison testing. *American Industrial Hygiene Association Journal* 59:862-870.

Federal Register. 1972. 30 CFR Part 11, 12, 13, 14 and 14a. *Federal Register* 37(59).

Frost and Sullivan Research Service. 2005. *U.S. markets for respiratory protection equipment—Analyst presentation.* http://www.frost.com/prod/servlet/report-brochure.pag?id=F160-01-00-00-00 (accessed March 26, 2008).

Gao, P., N. El-Ayouby, and J. T. Wassell. 2005. Change in permeation parameters and the decontamination efficacy of three chemical protective gloves after repeated exposures to solvents and thermal decontaminations. *American Journal of Industrial Medicine* 47:131-143.

Gardner, P., A. Richardson, K. Hofacre, and A. Rengasamy. 2006. *Efficiency of respirator filters against a viral aerosol.* Conference of the International Society for Respiratory Protection, August 28-31, Toronto, Canada.

IAFF (International Association of Fire Fighters). 2003. *PROJECT HEROES Homeland Emergency Response Operational and Equipment Systems, Task 1: A review of modern fire services hazards and protection needs.* Presentation to the National Personal Protective Technology Laboratory. http://www.cdc.gov/niosh/npptl/pdfs/ProjectHEROES.pdf (accessed March 17, 2008).

IOM (Institute of Medicine). 2006. *Reusability of facemasks during an influenza pandemic.* Washington, DC: The National Academies Press.

IOM. 2007. *Assessment of the NIOSH head-and-face anthropometric survey of U.S. respiratory users.* Washington, DC: The National Academies Press.

IOM. 2008. *Preparing for an influenza pandemic: Personal protective equipment for healthcare workers.* Washington, DC: The National Academies Press.

IOM and NRC (National Research Council). 2006. *Hearing loss research at NIOSH.* Committee to Review the NIOSH Hearing Loss Research Program. Rpt. No. 1, Reviews of Research Programs of the National Institute for Occupational Safety and Health. Washington, DC: The National Academies Press.

Jacobs Facilities, Inc. 2002. *Project development study for the National Personal Protective Technology Laboratory.* Final Document, April 2002.

Kim, S. C., M. S. Harrington, and D. Y. H. Pui. 2007. Experimental study of nanoparticles penetration through commercial filter media. *Journal of Nanoparticle Research* 9:117-125.

King, B. H., A. M. Ruminski, J. L. Snyder, and M. J. Sailor. 2007. Optical-fiber-mounted porous silicon photonic crystals for sensing organic vapor breakthrough in activated carbon. *Advanced Materials* 19(24):4530-4534.

LaTourrette, T., D. J. Peterson, J. T. Bartis, B. A. Jackson, and A. Houser. 2003. *Protecting emergency responders, Volume 2, Community views of safety and health risks and personal protection needs.* http://rand.org/pubs/monograph_reports/2005/MR1646.pdf (accessed March 17, 2008).

NIOSH. 2001. *Tracking occupational injuries, illnesses, and hazards: The NIOSH surveillance strategic plan.* http://www.cdc.gov/niosh/pdfs/2001-118.pdf (accessed March 19, 2008).

NIOSH. 2004a. *Program concept for total inward leakage (TIL) performance requirements and test methods.* http://www.cdc.gov/niosh/npptl/standardsdev/til/ (accessed March 5, 2008).

NIOSH. 2004b. *NIOSH respirator selection logic 2004.* http://www.cdc.gov/niosh/docs/2005-100/ (accessed March, 16, 2008).

NIOSH. 2004c. *Air-purifying escape hood respirators (escape hoods): Interim findings and guidance for models put into use prior to NIOSH CBRN Certification Standards.* http://www.cdc.gov/niosh/npptl/guidancedocs/interesc0404.html (accessed March 18, 2008).

NIOSH. 2005a. *Strategic plan for NIOSH nanotechnology research: Filling the knowledge gaps.* http://www.cdc.gov/niosh/topics/nanotech/strat_plan.html (accessed March 3, 2008).

NIOSH. 2005b. *Breakthrough 2004.* http://www.cdc.gov/niosh/docs/2005-125/ (accessed March 17, 2008).

NIOSH. 2005c. *CBRN APR interim guidance.* http://www.cdc.gov/niosh/npptl/guidancedocs/interesc0404.html (accessed March 18, 2008).

NIOSH. 2006. *Self-contained self-rescuer long term field evaluation: Combined eighth and ninth phase results.* http://www.cdc.gov/niosh/mining/pubs/pubreference/outputid2120.htm (accessed March 16, 2008).

NIOSH. 2007a. *NIOSH personal protective technology program: Evidence for the National Academies committee to review the NIOSH personal protective technology program.* Pittsburgh, PA: NIOSH.

NIOSH. 2007b. *PPT Program response to questions to NIOSH: Working Group 1.* Distributed to the Committee to Review the NIOSH Personal Protective Technology Program, November 14, 2007 (available through the National Academies Public Access File).

NIOSH. 2007c. *Certification application processing history, FY 2003-2007.* NIOSH response to inquiry regarding respirator certification numbers, December 13, 2007 (available through the National Academies Public Access File).

NIOSH. 2007d. *Approaches to safe nanotechnology.* http://www.cdc.gov/niosh/topics/nanotech/safenano/control.html (accessed March 4, 2008).

NIOSH. 2007e. *MultiVapor.* http://www.cdc.gov/niosh/npptl/multivapor/multivapor.html (accessed March 17, 2008).

NIOSH. 2007f. *Long-term field evaluation concept.* http://www.cdc.gov/niosh/review/public/NPPTL-LTFE/ (accessed March 17, 2008).

NIOSH. 2007g. *Final manufacturer/customer survey results.* http://www.cdc.gov/niosh/npptl/default.html (accessed March 18, 2008).

NIOSH. 2007h. *PPT Program response to questions to NIOSH: Working Group 3.* Distributed to the Committee to Review the NIOSH Personal Protective Technology Program, December 5, 2007 (available through the National Academies Public Access File).

NIOSH. 2008a. *Budget information on mining projects.* NIOSH response to committee questions, November 14, 2007 (available through the National Academies Public Access File).

NIOSH. 2008b. *Permeation calculator.* http://www.cdc.gov/niosh/npptl/PermeationCalculator/permeationcalc.html (accessed January 17, 2008).

NIOSH. 2008c. *Skin exposures and effects.* www.cdc.gov/niosh/topics/skin/ (accessed January 22, 2008).

NIOSH. 2008d. *PPT Program response to January 4, 2008 IOM request.* Distributed to the Committee to Review the NIOSH Personal Protective Technology Program, January 30, 2008 (available through the National Academies Public Access File).

NIOSH. 2008e. *PPT Program FTE summary.* Submitted by Maryann D'Alessandro via e-mail February 2, 2008. (available through the National Academies Public Access File).

NIOSH. 2008f. *NPPTL facial anthropometrics research roadmap.* http://www.cdc.gov/niosh/review/public/111/ (accessed March 4, 2008).

NIOSH. 2008g. *Personal protective equipment (PPE) for healthcare workers action plan.* http://www.cdc.gov/niosh/review/public/129/ (accessed March 5, 2008).

NIOSH. 2008h. *PPT surveillance program action plan. Draft, March 5, 2008* (available through the National Academies Public Access File).
NIOSH. 2008i. *Estimated timeline for 42 CFR Part 84 rulemaking, March 11, 2008* (available through the National Academies Public Access File).
NIOSH. 2008j. *Certified equipment list.* http://www.cdc.gov/niosh/npptl/topics/respirators/cel/ (accessed March 16, 2008).
NIOSH. 2008k. *CBRN respirator standards development.* http://www.cdc.gov/niosh/npptl/standardsdev/cbrn/default.html (accessed March, 17, 2008).
NIOSH. 2008l. *Office of Extramural Programs, grants process.* http://www.cdc.gov/niosh/oep/grants.html (accessed March 18, 2008).
NIOSH. 2008m. *Respirator testing.* http://www.cdc.gov/niosh/npptl/stps/Respirator_Testinghtm#STP_APR (accessed March 18, 2008).
NIOSH. 2008n. *Powered air-purifying respirator concept paper.* http://www.cdc.gov/niosh/npptl/resources/pressrel/letters/lttr-010308.html (accessed March 19, 2008).
NIOSH. 2008o. *Email from Maryann D'Alessandro,* March 26 (available through the National Academies Public Access File).
NIOSH. 2008p. *Fire Fighter Fatality Investigation and Prevention Program.* http://www.cdc.gov/niosh/fire/implweb.html (accessed April 7, 2008).
NIOSH. 2008q. *Program concept for total inward leakage (TIL) performance requirements and test methods.* http://www.cdc.gov/niosh/npptl/standardsdev/til/ (accessed March 19, 2008).
NPPTL (National Personal Protective Technology Laboratory). 2007. *Letter to all respirator manufacturers, Subject: Revised fees for CBRN respirator approvals, effective April 1, 2007.* http://www.cdc.gov/niosh/npptl/resources/pressrel/letters/lttr-031103b.html (accessed March 25, 2008).
NRC. 2007. *Measuring respirator use in the workplace.* Washington, DC: The National Academies Press.
NRC and IOM. 2007. *Mining safety and health research at NIOSH.* Committee to Review the NIOSH Mining Safety and Health Research Program. Rpt. No. 2, Reviews of Research Programs of the National Institute for Occupational Safety and Health. Washington, DC: The National Academies Press.
NRC and IOM. 2008a. *Agriculture, forestry, and fishing research at NIOSH.* Committee to Review the NIOSH Agriculture, Forestry, and Fishing Research Program. Rpt. No. 3, Reviews of Research Programs of the National Institute for Occupational Safety and Health. Washington, DC: The National Academies Press.
NRC and IOM. 2008b. *Respiratory disease research at NIOSH.* Committee to Review the NIOSH Respiratory Disease Research Program. Rpt. No. 4, Reviews of Research Programs of the National Institute for Occupational Safety and Health. Washington, DC: The National Academies Press.
Ramani, R., et al. 2003. *A compilation of personal protective equipment guidelines for emergency responders.* Pittsburgh, PA: NIOSH.
Rengasamy, S., R. Verbofsky, W. P. King, and R. Shaffer. 2007. Nanoparticle penetration through NIOSH-approved N95 filtering facepiece respirators. *Journal of the International Society for Respiratory Protection* 24:49-54.
Roberge, R. J. 2008a. Evaluation of the rationale for concurrent use of N95 filtering facepiece respirators with loose-fitting powered air-purifying respirators during aerosol-generating medical procedures. *American Journal of Infection Control* 36(2):135-141.
Roberge, R. J. 2008b. Effect of surgical masks worn concurrently over N95 filtering facepiece respirators: Extended service life versus increased user burden. *Journal of Public Health Management and Practice* 14(2):E19-E26.

Virginia Tech. 2005 *Advanced personal protective equipment: Challenges in protecting first responders.* http://www.cpe.vt.edu/appe/program.html (accessed January 22, 2008).

Vo, E. 2004. Application of colorimetric indicators and thermo-hand method to determine base permeation through chemical protective gloves. *Journal of Occupational and Environmental Hygiene* 1(12):799-805.

Wood, G. O. 2004. Estimating service lives of organic vapor respirator cartridges at all relative humidities. *Journal of Occupational and Environmental Hygiene* 1(7):472-492.

Wood, G. O. 2005. Estimating service lives of air-purifying respirator cartridges for reactive gas removal. *Journal of Occupational and Environmental Hygiene* 2(8):414-423.

Zhuang, Z., and B. Bradtmiller. 2005. Head-and-face anthropometric survey of U.S. respirator users. *Journal of Occupational and Environmental Hygiene* 2(11):567-576.

Zhuang, Z., B. Bradtmiller, and R. E. Shaffer. 2004. *New respirator fit test panels representing the current U.S. civilian workforce.* International Society for Respiratory Protection, November 9-12, Yokohama, Japan.

Zhuang, Z., L. M. Williams, D. J. Viscusi, and R. E. Shaffer. 2005. *Facial anthropometric differences among race/age groups.* American Industrial Hygiene Conference, May 23-26, Anaheim, CA.

Zhuang, Z., D. J. Viscusi, and A. Reddington. 2006. *Anthropometrics for developing headforms for testing respiratory and eye protective devices.* International Society for Respiratory Protection, August 27-September 1, Toronto, Canada.

Zhuang, Z., B. Bradtmiller, and R. Shaffer. 2007. New respirator fit test panels representing the current U.S. civilian workforce. *Journal of Occupational and Environmental Hygiene* 4:647-659.

3

Impact of the NIOSH PPT Program

Assessing the impact of public health efforts is always challenging. Trying to gauge to what extent disease or injury is prevented or is minimized usually involves assessing multiple potential causes and an array of individual and environmental influences. For most public health concerns, multiple preventive measures contribute to protection against injury or disease, and determining the extent of attribution of any one preventive measure or action is complex.

Quantitatively determining the extent to which personal protective technologies (PPT) contribute to worker well-being is a difficult matter. Engineering and administrative controls play a significant role in preventing hazardous exposures. Additionally, because the use of PPT is an individual-based measure, with effectiveness determined in large part by user decisions and quality of the fit, there can be wide variation in the apparent effectiveness of PPT products in preventing illness or injury. The many types of PPT products (e.g., respirators, protective clothing, hearing protection, eye protection, gloves, shoes, helmets, fall protection) and the fact that PPT is used in numerous occupational settings, each with its unique exposures and workplace demands, create a further challenge in attributing the impact of the National Institute for Occupational Safety and Health (NIOSH) PPT Program's efforts on improvements in worker safety and health.

This chapter begins with an appraisal of some of the external factors that affect the environment in which outcomes are attained. Several end outcomes are discussed in the chapter, with the focus of the text on the more tangible and identifiable intermediate outcomes of the PPT Program relevant to each of the major objectives. The chapter concludes with an overall assessment and scoring of the impact of the PPT Program.

EXTERNAL FACTORS

Determining the impact of the PPT Program[1] is affected by a number of external and underlying factors. A prime underlying factor is the congressional mandate stipulating NIOSH's responsibility to certify respirators. This chapter provides a more detailed discussion of the potential impacts of the certification mandate in providing the PPT Program with key oversight of the quality of respirators used in many U.S. worksites. The accompanying challenge, however, has been that respirator certification constitutes a significant percentage of the PPT Program's budget. Further, the congressional requirements for respirator certification place this function within the federal regulatory framework, which involves extensive procedures. Therefore, all changes to respirator certification regulations must go through a long process of federal rule making including publication, comment, and revision. This process ensures transparency to the general public but is time-intensive, particularly for dealing with products where the technology is evolving rapidly.

The short duration of time since the inception of the PPT Program is a key external factor. Respirator certification has been conducted at NIOSH since 1972, and research and standards-setting efforts were occurring in other NIOSH divisions before being transferred to the National Personal Protective Technology Laboratory (NPPTL). However, NPPTL was not founded until 2001, and therefore at the time of the writing of this report, barely seven years have elapsed. Given that the initial budgets in the early years of the laboratory were needed, to a large extent, for renovating the facilities, there have been only a few years on which to base an evaluation of the impact of the PPT Program. Further, NIOSH initiated the cross-sector PPT Program (NPPTL plus other PPT-relevant efforts) in 2005; this happened so recently that the PPT Program is just now having the opportunity to move beyond the initial organizational stages.

Also important to recognize is the impact and relevance of global events to the use of PPT. The terrorist attacks of 2001, the mine disasters of 2006, severe acute respiratory syndrome (SARS), and the widespread concern about the potential for an influenza pandemic have all contributed to heightening the public's awareness of PPT issues. These issues have all arisen amid the formative years of the PPT Program.

---

[1] As defined in Chapter 1, this report uses the term *PPT Program* to refer to the efforts from 2001 to the present that have been conducted by NIOSH relevant to the 12 PPT-relevant objectives that focus primarily on protection against respiratory and dermal hazards (Box 1-1).

END OUTCOMES

The majority of this chapter focuses on intermediate outcomes of the NIOSH PPT Program, because it is the intermediate outcomes that are more tangible and easier to quantify. However, the committee explored what could be said about the role of the PPT Program in impacting end outcomes, defined as reducing hazardous exposures and decreasing worker morbidity and mortality.

PPT products are used extensively in the U.S. workplace, and many PPT products have been found to be effective to varying degrees in reducing illness, injury, and death. As discussed in Chapter 1, estimates indicate that approximately 5 million U.S. workers are required to wear respirators in 1.3 million U.S. workplaces (OSHA, 2007).

In situations, such as firefighting, where conditions can be of immediate danger to life, PPT effectiveness can be seen every day in the survival and lack of harm experienced by most firefighters throughout the nation. In 2006, firefighters responded to 1,642,500 fire-related calls and suffered 44,210 injuries and 38 deaths due to operations at the fire site (NFPA, 2008a,b). A limited number of field studies of PPT have been conducted and provide evidence of the effectiveness of PPT products in the workplace. For example, a cohort of active firefighters in Boston followed for six years found that their longitudinal changes in pulmonary function were not correlated with a measure of firefighting exposure (Musk et al., 1982). Decrements in forced expiratory volume (FEV1) and forced vital capacity (FVC) were similar to levels in healthy nonsmoking adults. The authors attribute the lack of impact of long-term smoke exposure to increased use of PPT and to personnel selection factors. In a study of New York firefighters, researchers found that individuals who did not wear protective respiratory equipment had statistically significant decrements in acute pulmonary function (Brandt-Rauf et al., 1989). Similar results were found in a study of the effectiveness of respiratory protection for coal miners in West Virginia (Li et al., 2002). The researchers found a significant protective association between self-reported use of respirators and pulmonary function (FEV1). Recently, Banauch and colleagues (2006) studied more than 12,000 New York City firefighters and found that decline in respiratory functions (FVC and FEV1) between 1996 and 2001 were no different than in the general male population (annual decrease of 31 mL per year).

Protective clothing and hoods have also been found to reduce the incidence and severity of injuries due to burns experienced by firefighters. Rabbitts and colleagues (2005) found a reduction in hospitalizations of firefighters due to burn injuries from 53 patients per year to 15 patients per year during a 10-year time frame. Because the incidence of structural fires did not decline during that period, improvements in protective clothing were suggested as a plausible explanation for the decline. Prezant and colleagues (1999) found an 85 percent reduction in lower-extremity burn injuries, a 65 percent reduction in upper-extremity burn injuries, and a significant reduction in head burn injuries in New York City firefighters with the use of more protective uniforms and hoods.

In January 2006, miners in the Aracoma Alma Mine in West Virginia used NIOSH/MSHA-certified self-contained self-rescuer (SCSR) respirators, which chemically generate breathable oxygen, in their successful escape from a hazardous mixture of dense smoke and deadly concentrations of carbon monoxide after a mine fire (MSHA, 2006). This successful effort was presumably due in part to proper training as well as to the availability and maintenance of effective escape respirators. MSHA and the PPT Program worked closely in the Aracoma investigation to examine whether the escape respirators had been properly maintained and operable at the time of the fire.

Contributing to these positive end outcomes are manufacturers, work site managers, individual workers, federal and state agencies, research programs, organizations and associations that set product standards and certify product effectiveness, and many others. The NIOSH PPT Program is a critical component of this effort.

INTERMEDIATE OUTCOMES

Goal 1: Reduce Exposures to Inhalation Hazards

Although quantifying the impact of effective PPT on worker morbidity and mortality is challenging, a number of intermediate outcomes resulting from the work of the PPT Program point to progress. The major intermediate outcomes of the PPT Program are increases in the number of certified respirators, development and implementation of federal regulations and consensus standards, steps forward in increasing scientific knowledge regarding protection from inhalation hazards, and collaborations with other organizations and agencies.

Respirator Certification

Certified products The most significant outcome of the respirator certification program is an increase in the inventory of efficacious and reliable respirators for protection of workers from inhalation hazards. Since 2001, NIOSH has issued more than 1,600 respirator certifications (NIOSH, 2007a). NIOSH certification is the well-respected standard for asserting the efficacy of respirators. Both the Occupational Safety and Health Administration (OSHA) and the Mine Safety and Health Administration (MSHA) mandate that employers that have workers who may be exposed to respiratory hazards must use NIOSH-certified respirators (29 CFR 1910.34, 30 CFR 56.5005). Food and Drug Administration (FDA) approval of respirators for use in healthcare workplaces stipulates that the respirators must be certified by NIOSH (FDA, 2006). The Department of Homeland Security's (DHS) Authorized Equipment List also stipulates the use of NIOSH-certified respirators. Federal grants used to enhance the capacity of state and local jurisdictions to prevent or respond to crises require that respirators purchased under such grants be NIOSH CBRN (chemical, biological, radiological, and nuclear)-certified (DHS, 2008). NIOSH certification is also a requirement for respirators used in Quebec, Canada (NIOSH, 2007a), and the British Standards Institute has adopted requirements specified in the CBRN respirator test methods and other parts of the CBRN standard.

The actual inventory of NIOSH-certified respirators and respirator components in the United States is unknown to the committee. However, it is estimated that more than 5 million workers use respirators in the workplace. PPT Program staff members have reported a recent increase in applications for certification of N95 filtering facepiece respirators due to anticipated demand during an influenza pandemic (NIOSH, 2007a). The PPT Program is working to continue to improve its turnaround time in respirator certification with the goal of ensuring that the latest technology will be available for workers in the shortest reasonable time frame.

Dissemination of information Communication of information is critical to the impact of the PPT Program, which places great emphasis on disseminating information related to the respirator certification program via public meetings, user notices and concept papers posted online, or publication of guidance documents and fact sheets for users and manufacturers (see Chapter 2). The dissemination of user notices of respirator certification recissions, recalls, or retrofits is particularly critical to ensuring that workers have effective equipment. The PPT Program has developed an extensive capacity to reach stakeholders through its listserv with updates on relevant research, policy and standards, and respirator certification activities (NIOSH, 2008b). There are more than 2,500 listserv subscribers representing users, manufacturers, and stakeholders from 30 countries. Efforts have also been made by the PPT Program to provide a central online information resource site to respirator manufacturers with links to the certification application procedures, standard test procedures, Certified Equipment List, archives of letters to manufacturers, and respirator user notices (NIOSH, 2008c).

Other organizations are also disseminating information on NIOSH certification to the user community. For example, the Responder Knowledge Base (RKB) provides information to first responders (RKB, 2008). Sponsored by DHS, and in conjunction with the InterAgency Board for Equipment Standardization and Interoperability (IAB) and many partner organizations and agencies including NIOSH, the RKB is an online database of products that are in compliance with existing standards. The goal is an authoritative resource for equipment selection.

Products in the RKB are closely related to the DHS Authorized Equipment List (DHS, 2008) and the IAB's Selected Equipment List, both of which specify NIOSH-certified CBRN respirators and compliance with NIOSH CBRN standards.

Federal Regulations

Respirators are the only type of PPT that is federally certified (42 CFR 84). Federal regulations stipulate the specific test procedures and performance criteria for certification. Although updating the regulations through the federal rule-making process is a lengthy undertaking (see Chapter 2), once they have been finalized the PPT Program can implement the changes rapidly and use the revisions to further refine subsequent respirator certifications.

The PPT Program's work in the promulgation of CBRN regulations for respirator certification has had considerable impact on ensuring that these highly specialized respirators meet specific criteria to offer effective protection to emergency workers and others with the potential for exposure. The Department of Homeland Security and the IAB have adopted the NIOSH CBRN respirator standards (IAB, 2007). National Fire Protection Association (NFPA) standards (NFPA 1500, 1991, and 1994) require NIOSH CBRN certification for self-contained breathing apparatus and air-purifying respirators. Internationally, the NIOSH CBRN respirator standards performance requirement and test methods have been incorporated by the British Standards Institute (NIOSH, 2007a). These achievements have been the result of activities that cut across the PPT Program. For example, as a result of the anthropometric research program, head and neck circumference data were used as a basis for the new NIOSH standard for CBRN escape respirators or hoods.

Other federal regulatory standards are in various stages of development (see Chapter 2), and their implementation needs to be accelerated to the extent feasible under federal rule making. Proposed changes to the federal regulations, including tests of total inward leakage, could yield improved testing procedures and improved respirator performance if implemented.

Consensus Standards

The committee draft of the new International Organization for Standardization (ISO) specification standard (ISO 16976-2 *Respiratory Protective Devices: Human Factors, Part 2: Anthropometrics*) incorporates the findings of the initial PPT Program studies. PPT Program findings are also being used to establish the parameters for standardized headforms for respirator testing.

The work that went into preparation of the *Approaches to Safe Nanotechnology* document (NIOSH, 2007c) by NIOSH has been incorporated into draft ISO and

ASTM International standards that are working their way through those organizations. The PPT Program has also proposed a new work item to the ASTM F23.40 Subcommittee based on the work done on viral decontamination (*Test Method for Evaluation of the Effectiveness of Biological Decontamination Procedures on Viral Contaminated Air Permeable Material*).

Scientific Knowledge and Technology Transfer

The various and disparate activities bundled together under the PPT respiratory protection research program have, individually and collectively, resulted in significant advances in protection against respiratory hazards and exposures. The science that drives those advances is associated largely with the amount of resources devoted to the enterprise as well as the amount of time in which the PPT Program has been able to focus on the topic. For example, the contributions to scientific knowledge of the high-priority, decade-old program to develop CBRN respirator standards has clearly placed the PPT Program in a leadership role, and this leadership has played out in leading-edge contributions to national and international standards-development organizations. On the other hand, more recent—and less generously funded—projects to quantify the impact of PPE on viral transmission and to evaluate respiratory protection against nanoparticles are in the early phases of research, and the scope of the PPT Program's role in this area is still being explored. Projects to ensure the availability of improved mine emergency respirators, improve the reliability and level of protection of PPT by designs that better fit the users, and develop end-of-service-life indicator (ESLI) technologies have produced important, identifiable scientific advances although their promise still lies in the future.

The PPT Program's work on improving mine escape respirators is being accomplished through efforts to explore new technologies, revise federal regulatory standards, and learn from field evaluations. This is a priority area for the PPT Program, but one in which resources are fairly limited (see Chapter 2). As noted above, NIOSH-certified SCSR respirators were instrumental in the safe rescue of miners in a West Virginia mine fire in 2006. Efforts to improve SCSR respirators are ongoing with a focus on developing technologies to provide an increased supply of breathable air that is accessible through multiple points along an escape route. The PPT Program is in the midst of expanding its Long-Term Field Evaluation of the emergency respirators to ensure a large enough sample for achieving statistical significance and to document corrective actions needed (NIOSH, 2007b). The PPT Program is working with a private-sector contractor to develop and test a prototype for a new dockable SCSR with the goal of extending the protection offered by these devices in the event of a disaster. The PPT Program has worked with MSHA to refine training materials for SCSRs that include video- and computer-based training focused on improving the efforts of mine workers in inspecting, maintaining, and using the respirators; the training modules have been distributed to more than 1,800 mines (NIOSH, 2007a).

Studies in the laboratory have demonstrated the efficacy of respirators (for example, Coffey and colleagues, 1998a,b). The PPT Program's research on improving respirator fit by beginning to examine total inward leakage (TIL) and utilizing anthropometric data will contribute significantly to scientific knowledge in this field through the development of new technologies and enhanced analytic methods. As recommended in the Institute of Medicine report on this research area (IOM, 2007) and further developed in the PPT Program's action plan on anthropometric research (NIOSH, 2008a), there are a number of ways to continue to refine research in this area. Also, as described in Chapter 4, the PPT Program has some initial plans to explore advances in materials sciences and other disciplines that may eventually lead to a respirator that fits all face shapes and sizes without the need for fit testing.

The PPT Program's research on viral transmission and protection in the event of pandemic influenza is still in the early phases but is pursuing answers to important questions. PPT Program research in this area has resulted in further understanding of respirator decontamination, and efforts are under way to learn more about the viability of the influenza virus on PPT equipment. PPT Program scientists have provided their expertise to relevant national and international efforts on PPT and pandemic influenza, including a review of the U.S. national implementation plan at the request of the Homeland Security Council and input to the World Health Organization regarding the revision of its recommendations for respiratory protection during a pandemic (NIOSH, 2007a).

The work on nanotechnology has had some early impact that sets the stage for further advances in the science. NIOSH and the DuPont Occupational Safety and Health Consortium have a memorandum of understanding (MOU) focused on work to examine test methods regarding the performance of protective clothing and respirators exposed to nanoparticles. Ongoing work with the Center for Filtration Research at the University of Minnesota is also focused on respirator filtration efficiency against nanoparticles.

The ESLI research program has made important contributions to worker safety by developing software models (distributed through OSHA's website) that are used by employers to predict the service life of respirator cartridges. Previously, odor detection of gases or vapors by workers had been one of the methods used for determining service life. The OSHA requirement for a more accurate method (OSHA, 2008) and the PPT Program's development of the *MultiVapor* and *Breakthrough* software (see Chapter 2) have improved the ability of employers to better protect workers from exposures to hazardous chemicals. The recent release of revised software allows temperature and humidity to be factored into the model and allows for consideration of chemical mixtures. The PPT Program needs to continue to make the models as user-friendly as possible and to continue to work with OSHA and employers to publicize the availability of the model.

The ESLI sensor project to develop technology for incorporating sensors into respirator cartridges to determine their lifetime has a significant potential impact for all industries. This sensor technology measures the capacity of the cartridge or canister during use and alerts the user when the cartridge needs to be changed. The indicator can be an audio or a visual display and has numerous potential applications in many industries because the technology is not contaminant-specific. The PPT Program is currently working with a group of manufacturers to test the sensor technology in a variety of simulated workplaces.

Collaborations

The PPT Program's work on expediting the development of standards specific to CBRN respirators was based on extensive collaborations. Efforts began in 1999 with discussions at a workshop sponsored by NIOSH, the Department of Defense, and OSHA (NIOSH, 2007a). Early on, it was determined that the CBRN respirator standards development effort would also involve NFPA and the National Institute of Standards and Technology (NIST). Memoranda of understanding were put in place that defined each agency's role, and the PPT Program worked extensively with these agencies as well as many others (including respirator manufacturers) to specify the hazards, define the operational requirements, and determine the protection requirements and standards.

The PPT Program provided technical assistance to the Food and Drug Administration in efforts to develop the new classification for respirators for the general public in the event of pandemic influenza (FDA, 2007). Further, the PPT Program has actively sponsored and participated in workshops on the topic of PPT for an influenza pandemic. These efforts include a January 2006 NIOSH conference *Public Use of Respiratory Protection* and a joint U.S. Department of Agriculture (USDA)-FDA-NIOSH interagency workgroup on PPT and other issues relevant to avian influenza in the workplace (NIOSH, 2007a). Research efforts to examine biocidal technologies and their use in respirators have involved developing MOUs with six respirator manufacturers. Collaborations with the Department of Veterans Affairs are focused on examining issues of comfort and wearability (NIOSH, 2007a).

The PPT Program's research into developing software models to predict the end of service life for respirator cartridges has involved multiple partners including the American Chemistry Council, the International Safety Equipment Association,

Los Alamos National Laboratory, the National Paint and Coatings Association, and others. More recent research efforts focused on the development of sensor-based approaches (to be embedded in the cartridge) are part of an active collaboration with the Microelectrical Systems Laboratory of Carnegie Mellon University and the U.S. Air Force. The current prototype system has been refined through five iterations of sensor design. Based on this collaborative research, the PPT Program has moved from basic research, to development of the sensor system, to actively working with manufacturers on testing these devices integrated into commercial respirators.

As a part of the recent nanotechnology efforts, the PPT Program has collaborated extensively with other NIOSH colleagues in efforts to develop and implement the NIOSH strategic plan. Finally, the PPT Program works with MSHA to update the materials used to train miners in donning SCSR respirators.

Committee's Comments on Impact on Occupational Safety and Health

As noted above, the NIOSH respirator certification program impacts worker safety by ensuring a reliable inventory of respirators for protection against respiratory hazards. Respirator manufacturers depend on NIOSH certification to independently evaluate the performance and quality of the products that they sell to employers.

Further, the PPT Program's efforts to reduce illnesses or injuries due to inhalation hazards can be seen through contributions to the development of standards, regulations, and research. However, the program's impact could be even greater. Areas in which the impact of the respirator certification program could be improved include the following:

- *Registration of devices:* The respirator certification and respirator purchasing processes do not currently have provisions for registering the purchase of respirators. As a result, neither NIOSH nor manufacturers have a direct method for contacting employers who purchased respirators with notices indicating that a problem or recall has occurred. MSHA has recently begun requiring registration of SCSRs by mine operators.
- *Field testing of certified respirators:* Field tests of certified respirators are needed to ensure that these products perform effectively in the workplace.
- *Comparability of certification test results:* Increasing the amount of certification testing data provided online will allow purchasers, particularly employers, to learn more about these results and to compare products.

- *Expedited revisions of certification regulations:* As detailed in Chapter 2, much needs to be done to ensure that federal regulations are updated to incorporate state-of-the-art technologies into the respirator certification process.

The inhalation research program has begun to make significant contributions to worker protection from inhalation hazards in that it informs the certification program, provides information to manufacturers and employers that can assist in development of better protective equipment, and enables formulation of standards, both in the United States and abroad, that underpin inhalation PPT programs. In selecting the objectives for research programs to reduce exposure to inhalation hazards, NIOSH has appropriately focused on key issues of interest to the community, such as pandemic influenza, as well as more specific projects to improve equipment (mine emergency respirators), add reliability (anthropometric fit), and ensure the continued effectiveness of equipment in the hands of users (end-of-service-life indicators).

As these research programs move from basic to applied sciences, new questions have arisen and new avenues of investigation have opened. For example, the work on influenza virus protection has shown that the N95 disposable protective masks can prevent inhalation of the virus, but new questions about the ability of other types of equipment to protect against influenza have now been raised. In addition, there are questions related to reusability that require answers as to whether respirators once exposed to influenza can become infectious fomites for contagion. If so, reusability could not occur without an effective decontamination protocol. If not, reusability and a shift toward personal nondisposable respirators would make economic sense during a pandemic.

Goal 2: Reduce Exposures to Dermal Hazards

Although the NIOSH PPT Program does not certify PPT related to dermal exposures, intermediate outcomes of relevance include increases in scientific knowledge, technology transfer, and development of consensus standards.

Scientific Knowledge and Technology Transfer

The dermal component of PPT research at NIOSH is a relatively new addition to the portfolio and one that receives limited amounts of funding (approximately $765,000 in FY 2007; NIOSH, 2007a). However, even within these constraints, the PPT Program has advanced the scientific methodology and knowledge base on dermal protection. One of the important outcomes of PPT Program research in this area has been the development of novel test protocols. As discussed below the research protocol developed by PPT Program staff in their work on testing firefighter ensembles is becoming a standard test method and can bring some consistency and comparability to PPE ensemble testing. Similarly, the stored thermal energy test apparatus, developed through research funded by the PPT Program, is being used for the interlaboratory testing conducted under the auspices of the NFPA Research Foundation through grants from DHS.

The PPT Program's work on cumulative permeation dermal risk assessment is a major step forward in addressing the many unknowns in this understudied area. Currently this research is largely confined to chemical warfare agents. However, it has potential for much broader impact when resources become available to expand the research focus to include protection against the many, and much more common, toxic industrial chemicals found in the workplace.

The establishment of physiological assessment facilities increases the national capacity for assessing these important performance attributes. Although the physiology laboratory is relatively new (established in 2005), this research facility offers the potential for significant contributions to the development of effective PPT that is less physiologically stressful and therefore easier for workers to tolerate.

Physiologic and ergonomic studies conducted by the PPT Program have been an important part of Project HEROES® (Homeland Emergency Response Operational and Equipment Systems), an effort designed to advance the technology of CBRN structural firefighting ensembles (IAFF, 2008). Researchers evaluated the effects of incorporated designs on the physiological burden of the turn-out gear developed by Project HEROES. Some of these advances included expansion of protective capabilities (CBRN), an innovative moisture barrier and gasket technologies, advanced outer materials, and cooling systems for the upper torso.

Although it is typically difficult to document the impact of forward strides in a rapidly evolving area of scientific knowledge, research conducted by the PPT Program often has applicability to the testing and development of protective gear. These efforts have provided inputs to product specifications and ASTM International and NFPA standards revisions. Field assessments of chemical protective clothing, gloves, and other types of dermal and injury-related PPT would be particularly helpful in broadening our understanding of these important and understudied areas (see further discussion in Chapters 4 and 5).

Consensus Standards

The PPT Program has made significant contributions to furthering standards relevant to protective clothing and other dermal protection. Through staff participation in ASTM and NFPA technical committees and the supporting research efforts necessary to inform these efforts, the PPT Program has provided the information and expertise necessary to move forward on a number of new test methods and performance standards for PPT relevant to protective clothing and equipment (Table 3-1). Of particular note are NFPA 1971 and NFPA 1999. PPT Program personnel played key roles in the 2007 edition of NFPA 1971, *Standard on Protective Ensembles for Structural Fire Fighting and Proximity Fire Fighting*. Their efforts greatly assisted the development of the optional CBRN requirements. Additionally, the PPT Program has worked on the test methodology as well as the product evaluations for the revision of NFPA 1999, *Standard on Protective Clothing for Emergency Medical Operations*. Further, the PPT Program sought input from a number of focus groups on this topic (NIOSH, 2007a). Overall, recent efforts by the PPT Program have contributed significantly to seven NFPA and two ASTM standards.

TABLE 3-1 Recent Consensus Standards with PPT Program Involvement

Date	Standard
2005	NFPA 1991, Standard on Vapor-Protective Ensembles for Hazardous Materials Emergencies (2005 Edition)
2005	NFPA 1992, Standard on Liquid Splash-Protective Ensembles and Clothing for Hazardous Materials Emergencies (2005 Edition)
2007	PPT Program Physiological Protocol approved as an ASTM International standard practice for physiological evaluation of protective ensembles based on research conducted in the PPT Program laboratory
2007	ASTM F2588-06 Standard Test Method for Man-in-Simulant Test for Protective Ensembles
2007	NFPA 1951, Standard on Protective Ensemble for Technical Rescue Operations (2007 Edition)
2007	NFPA 1971, Standard on Protective Ensembles for Structural Fire Fighting and Proximity Fire Fighting (2007 Edition)
2007	NFPA 1994, Standard on Protective Ensembles for First Responders to CBRN Terrorism Incidents (2007 Edition)
2008	NFPA 1851, Standard on Selection, Care and Maintenance of Structural Fire Fighting Protective Ensembles (2007 Edition)
2008	NFPA 1999, Standard on Protective Clothing for Emergency Medical Operations (2008 Edition)

NOTE: ASTM = ASTM International (formerly, the American Society for Testing and Materials); NFPA = National Fire Protection Association.

The permeation calculator, developed through PPT Program research and analysis, is in the process of being incorporated into at least two ASTM standards as a tool for the calculation of permeation parameters from laboratory-based permeation test results. The calculated parameters are used to select appropriate chemical protective clothing based on permeation resistance. As mentioned above, the protocol developed by the PPT Program for testing prototype firefighter ensembles through Project HEROES has recently been approved as Standard Physiology Test Practice (ASTM 23.60). This protocol sets the stage for further work on improving the ensembles by providing a consistent approach to testing and thus constitutes an important intermediate outcome that will require manufacturers to provide ensembles of equal protection. A valid and consistent testing method will enhance the reliability of the research-to-practice and technology transfer efforts.

A number of stakeholders who spoke to the committee at its December 2007 workshop emphasized the valued contributions of PPT Program staff in providing leadership and expertise to a number of standards-development committees. One person noted that what previously had been a fairly passive level of involvement by PPT Program staff has now changed into an active contributory role.

As seen in Table 3-1, PPT ensembles are a focus of efforts in standards setting. The committee strongly urges continued efforts to expand work on developing integrated PPT components. In the committee's view, one of the efforts most needed in this field is progress toward protective equipment that is interchangeable, provides full coverage, and is consistent with ergonomics and human factors principles related to usability (see Chapters 4 and 5).

PPT Program efforts also contribute to resources used by employers and employees. One of the outcomes of the PPT Program's decontamination research is a contribution to the content of the American Industrial Hygiene Association (AIHA) guideline *Decontamination of Chemical Protective Clothing and Equipment* (AIHA, 2005). A PPT Program staff member, at the request of AIHA, served as the lead facilitator of the guideline development effort. The PPT Program also worked with AIHA to support research-to-practice activities by developing recommendations for user practice.

Committee's Comments on Impact on Occupational Safety and Health

Given the limited resources available for work on dermal PPT, the PPT Program has had, and continues to have, considerable impact. Foremost among the intermediate outcomes are the consensus standards that are developed and approved with substantive input from PPT Program staff and, in many cases, through research conducted or funded by the PPT Program. These standards provide the criteria for producing and testing high-quality and effective PPT. Recent efforts have focused on emergency responders, but with increased resources, similar steps forward could be taken on PPT for agricultural workers, healthcare workers, construction workers, and those in other occupations where the prevalence of toxic exposures and the large number of workplaces make this an important public health consideration.

Goal 3: Reduce Exposures to Injury Hazards

As discussed in Chapter 2, the committee was asked to look at only one PPT objective relevant to injury—the personal alert safety system (PASS) alarms that identify the location of a worker in distress. Work is in progress at NIOSH on PPT relevant to other injury hazards, particularly hearing loss, fall protection, and vibration protection. Those issues do not fall under the purview of this report but should be incorporated into the overall efforts of the expanded PPT Program discussed in Chapter 5.

Work by the PPT Program and other NIOSH divisions through the investigation of firefighter fatalities contributed to an alert published by NFPA focused on the potential failure of PASS alarm signals to operate at high temperatures (NFPA, 2007). PPT Program staff participated on the NFPA technical committee that revised the performance requirements. The resulting 2007 revised NFPA standard increased the temperatures and water immersion criteria used for testing these devices. Although this is currently a focused and limited area of ongoing effort in the PPT Program, there is great potential for further work on protective sensor technology (see Chapter 4).

Surveillance

The PPT Program's surveillance efforts to date have focused on the use and dissemination of results of the 2001 NIOSH-Bureau of Labor Statistics (BLS) survey of respirator usage. The survey results were published in *Respirator Usage in Private Sector Firms* (BLS and NIOSH, 2003) and represent an advance in the nation's understanding of employer practices with regard to respirator use as of 2001 (NRC, 2007). The survey's findings were used extensively for the analysis of the regulatory impact of the proposed assigned protection factor (APF) rule of the OSHA 1910.134 respiratory protection standard (Steelnack, 2007). Also, as noted in the PPT Program's evidence package, the survey enabled NIOSH, OSHA, and MSHA to better target workplace educational and information programs (NIOSH, 2007a). One key finding that a large number of establishments had airline respirator hose couplings compatible with other air or gas supply lines led OSHA to issue the Safety and Health Information Bulletin *Deaths Involving the Inadvertent Connection of Air-line Respirators to Inert Gas Supplies* (OSHA, 2004).

Several issues that limited the usefulness of the survey were reported in the NIOSH-sponsored National Research Council (NRC) report *Measuring Respirator Use in the Workplace* (NRC, 2007). The NRC report contained a number of recommendations for future survey and other surveillance activities and has had the positive impact of assisting in the development of a PPT Surveillance Program Action Plan (NIOSH, 2008d). This plan, available to the committee in draft form, specifies a number of short- and long-range activities for PPT surveillance to systematically use data as an input to program decisions. In its draft form, the plan calls for the following:

- A management framework that will closely align program mission, goals, and objectives with surveillance activities
- A focus on PPT use and nonuse; defects, recalls, claims, and complaints; and information about injuries, illnesses, and deaths related to improper PPT design or use
- An ongoing nationwide PPT survey conducted in each of the eight National Occupational Research Agenda (NORA) industry sectors,[2] with one to three sectors (depending on size) surveyed each year
- Special surveys conducted either as a supplement to the ongoing survey or independent from the ongoing survey to gather information on emerging issues, special needs, and specific study questions
- Other data collection and analysis activities that will be based on secondary data sources, other databases, literature searches, and such activities as focus groups, panels, and field observations—these activities would include developing an ongoing Demonstration and Sentinel Surveillance System for monitoring PPT-related efforts in five major hospitals; integration of the Long-Term Field Evaluation program of self-contained self-rescuers for miners into the surveillance program; and examination of other data sources, such as the Fire Fighter Fatality Investigation and Prevention Program, the National Electronic Injury Surveillance System, and the Sentinel Event Notification System for Occupational Risks
- A research-to-practice plan to support these collection and analysis activities

The draft timeline for implementing this plan envisions an ongoing examination of secondary data sources, the conduct of special studies beginning in FY

---

[2]The NORA industry sectors are Agriculture, Forestry, and Fishing; Construction; Healthcare and Social Assistance; Manufacturing; Mining; Services; Transportation, Warehousing and Utilities; and Wholesale and Retail Trade.

2008, and a several-year buildup to the collection of the first sectoral surveillance surveys in FY 2011. The committee applauds the efforts of the PPT Program to bring scientific rigor to PPT surveillance, but remains concerned about acquisition of the resources required for such an undertaking. Further, the committee urges PPT surveillance efforts to focus on all types of PPT.

OVERALL ASSESSMENT OF IMPACT

NIOSH is nationally and internationally recognized for its respirator certification program. OSHA and MSHA require that the respirators used in U.S. workplaces be NIOSH-certified. The PPT Program also took a leadership role in developing and expediting federal regulatory standards for CBRN respirators. This effort involved extensive collaboration with multiple federal agencies, manufacturers, and professional associations (see Chapter 2). For example, OSHA and NIOSH collaboratively developed a CBRN PPT Selection Matrix for Emergency Responders (OSHA, 2005).

Impacts on reducing hazardous exposures or preventing illness or injury are difficult to attribute directly to the work of a single federal agency. However because the PPT Program certifies that respirators meet a number of rigorous, pre-specified performance criteria, the committee felt justified in acknowledging that positive end outcomes have occurred that are attributable to the PPT Program's role in respirator certification. For workers who have few other protections from hazardous workplace exposures, such as firefighters, the value of effective PPT is a daily reality. As noted above, successful mine escapes have occurred because miners had access to effective respirators that prevented exposure to lethal levels of carbon monoxide. Having such equipment in place involves the collaborative efforts of manufacturers, professional associations, employers, employees, unions, state and federal agencies, and many others. However, the committee recognizes the central and vital role that the PPT Program plays in this effort.

Important intermediate outcomes also appear to be the result of active participation by PPT Program staff members in consensus standards-development efforts. The PPT Program has leveraged its limited resources well in its participation in national and international consensus standards organizations. Several recent ISO and ASTM International standards have incorporated test methods developed through PPT Program research. The PPT Program staff has also led or been instrumental in research on a number of key issues, although, as in several other important areas, budget restraints substantially limit the extent of research efforts. Work on protection against viral transmission (particularly related to pandemic influenza) and on nanotechnology is in the early phases and has not yet received the resources or had the opportunity to produce intermediate outcomes.

The committee believes that although great strides have been made in improving respirators, much could be done to address other types of PPT (e.g., protective clothing, protective eyewear, gloves, hearing protection, hard hats, fall harnesses) with additional resources. Additionally, the successful focus on improving PPT for emergency responders now needs to be expanded to other occupations, including agricultural workers, construction workers, healthcare workers, and industrial workers, where the public health impact is likely to be far more substantial. Work on protective ensembles also holds great promise, and innovative approaches need to be developed to provide seamless interfaces among different types and components of PPT.

As discussed in Chapter 2, the committee urges expedited efforts to revise federal certification regulations, so that new technologies and testing methodologies can be utilized to improve the efficacy of respirators and allow for innovation in the design and function of this equipment. Similarly, there is much that should be done to improve protective clothing, eyewear, gloves, and other types of PPT, contingent upon additional resources.

On the basis of its review of the PPT Program's work in research, respirator certification, and policy and standards setting, the committee has assigned the NIOSH Personal Protective Technology Program a score of 4 for impact. This score, according to the scoring criteria outlined by the framework committee, reflects the judgment that the PPT Program has made probable contributions to end outcomes in addition to well-accepted intermediate outcomes (see Box 3-1 and Appendix A). In the judgment of the committee, the program could further improve its impact score by applying the lessons learned in the development of CBRN respirator standards to other types of PPT (e.g., protective clothing, protective eyewear, gloves)

BOX 3-1
Scoring Criteria for Impact

5 = The program has made major contribution(s) to worker health and safety on the basis of end outcomes or well-accepted intermediate outcomes.
4 = The program has made some contributions to end outcomes or well-accepted intermediate outcomes.
3 = The program's activities are ongoing, and outputs are produced that are likely to result in improvements in worker health and safety (with explanation of why not rated higher). Well-accepted outcomes have not been recorded.
2 = The program's activities are ongoing, and outputs are produced that may result in new knowledge or technology, but only limited application is expected. Well-accepted outcomes have not been recorded.
1 = Activities and outputs do not result in or are NOT likely to have any application.

and emphasizing development and testing of protective ensembles and other integrated approaches to PPT.

REFERENCES

AIHA (American Industrial Hygiene Association) Protective Clothing Committee. 2005. *Guidelines for the decontamination of chemical protective clothing and equipment.* Fairfax, VA: AIHA Press.

Banauch, G. I., C. Hall, M. Weiden, H. W. Cohen, T. K. Aldrich, V. Christodoulou, N. Arcentales, K. J. Kelly, and D. J. Prezant. 2006. Pulmonary function after exposure to the World Trade Center collapse in the New York City Fire Department. *American Journal of Respiratory and Critical Care Medicine* 174:312-319.

BLS (Bureau of Labor Statistics) and NIOSH (National Institute for Occupational Safety and Health). 2003. *Respirator usage in private sector firms, 2001.* Washington, DC: BLS and NIOSH.

Brandt-Rauf, P. W., B. Cosman, L. F. Fallon, Jr., T. Tarantini, and C. Idema. 1989. Health hazards of firefighters: Acute pulmonary effects after toxic exposures. *British Journal of Industrial Medicine* 46(3):209-211.

Coffey, C. C., D. L. Campbell, W. R. Myers, Z. Zhuang, and S. Das. 1998a. Comparison of six respirator fit test methods with an actual measurement of exposure in a simulated health-care environment: Part I—Protocol development. *American Industrial Hygiene Association Journal* 59:852-861.

Coffey, C. C., D. L. Campbell, W. R. Myers, Z. Zhuang, and S. Das. 1998b. Comparison of six respirator fit test methods with an actual measurement of exposure in a simulated health-care environment: Part II—Method comparison testing. *American Industrial Hygiene Association Journal* 59:862-870.

DHS (Department of Homeland Security). 2008. *Authorized equipment list.* http://www.ojp.usdoj.gov/odp/grants_equipment.htm (accessed March 19, 2008).

FDA (Food and Drug Administration). 2006. *FDA's role in regulating PPE.* http://www.fda.gov/cdrh/ppe/fdarole.html (accessed April 2, 2008).

FDA. 2007. *Respirators for public health emergencies.* http://www.fda.gov/consumer/updates/respirators061107.html (accessed June 2, 2008).

IAB (InterAgency Board for Equipment Standardization and Interoperability). 2007. *Selected equipment list.* http://www.iab.gov/Documents.aspx (accessed March 17, 2008).

IAFF (International Association of Fire Fighters). 2008. *Project HEROES.* http://www.iaf.org/hs/Project%20HEROES.htm (accessed April 8, 2008).

IOM (Institute of Medicine). 2007. *Assessment of the NIOSH head-and-face anthropometric survey of U.S. respirator users.* Washington, DC: The National Academies Press.

Li, H., M. L. Wang, N. Seixas, A. Ducatman, and E. L. Petsonk. 2002. Respiratory protection: Associated factors and effectiveness of respirator use among underground coal miners. *American Journal of Industrial Medicine* 42(1):55-62.

MSHA (Mine Safety and Health Administration). 2006. *Aracoma Coal Company, Inc., Aracoma Alma Mine #1. Fatal mine fire.* http://www.msha.gov/FATALS/2006/ARACOMA/ARACOMAREPORT.ASP (accessed March 10, 2008).

Musk, A. W., J. W. Peters, L. Bernstein, C. Rubin, and C. B. Monroe. 1982. Pulmonary function in firefighters: A six-year follow-up in the Boston Fire Department. *American Journal of Industrial Medicine* 3(1):3-9.

NFPA (National Fire Protection Association). 2007. *PASS performance issues addressed in new edition of NFPA standard, NFPA Alert Notice Update, February 9, 2007.* http://www.nfpa.org/itemDetail.asp?categoryID=823&itemID=26606&cookie%5Ftest=1 (accessed March 26, 2008).

NFPA. 2008a. *The U.S. Fire Service, 2006.* http://www.nfpa.org/categoryList.asp?categoryID=955& URL=Research%20&%20Reports/Fire%20statistics/The%20U.S.%20fire%20service (accessed March 26, 2008).

NFPA. 2008b. *The U.S. Fire Service, fire department calls.* http://www.nfpa.org/itemDetail.asp?categoryID=955&itemID=23850&URL=Research%20&%20Reports/Fire%20statistics/The%20U.S.%20fire%20service (accessed March 26, 2008).

NIOSH. 2007a. *NIOSH personal protective technology program: Evidence for the National Academies committee to review the NIOSH personal protective technology program.* Pittsburgh, PA: NIOSH.

NIOSH. 2007b. *Long-term field evaluation concept.* http://www.cdc.gov/niosh/review/public/NPPTL-LTFE/ (accessed March 17, 2008).

NIOSH. 2007c. *Approaches to safe nanotechnology.* http://www.cdc.gov/hiosh/topics/nanotech/safenano/control.html (accessed March 4, 2008).

NIOSH. 2008a. *NPPTL facial anthropometrics research roadmap.* http://www.cdc.gov/niosh/review/public/111/ (accessed March 4, 2008).

NIOSH. 2008b. *Email listserv.* http://www.cdc.gov/niosh/npptl/sub-NPPTL.html (accessed March 19, 2008).

NIOSH. 2008c. *Certification program support for manufacturers.* http://www.cdc.gov/niosh/npptl/resources/certpgmspt/ (accessed March 19, 2008).

NIOSH. 2008d. *PPT surveillance program action plan. Draft, March 5, 2008.* (accessible through the National Academies Public Access File).

NRC (National Research Council). 2007. *Measuring respirator use in the workplace.* Washington, DC: The National Academies Press.

OSHA (Occupational Safety and Health Administration). 2004. *Deaths involving the inadvertent connection of air-line respirators to inert gas supplies.* http://www.osha.gov/dts/shib/shib042704.html (accessed March 20, 2008).

OSHA. 2005. *OSHA/NIOSH interim guidance—April 1, 2005. Chemical-biological-radiological-nuclear (CBRN). Personal protective equipment selection matrix for emergency responders.* http://www.osha.gov/SLTC/emergencypreparedness/cbrnmatrix/index.html (accessed March 17, 2008).

OSHA. 2007. *Safety and health topics: Respiratory protection.* http://www.osha.gov/SLTC/respiratoryprotection/ (accessed March 12, 2008).

OSHA. 2008. *Respirator change schedules.* http://www.osha.gov/SLTC/etools/respiratory/change_schedule.html (accessed March 17, 2008).

Prezant, D. J., K. J. Kelly, K. S. Malley, M. L. Karwa, M. T. McLaughlin, R. Hirschorn, and A. Brown. 1999. Impact of a modern firefighting protective uniform on the incidence and severity of burn injuries in New York City firefighters. *Journal of Occupational and Environmental Medicine* 41(6):469-479.

Rabbitts, A., N. E. Alden, M. Scalabrino, and R. W. Yurt. 2005. Outpatient firefighter burn injuries: A 3-year review. *Journal of Burn Care and Rehabilitation* 26(4):348-351.

RKB (Responder Knowledge Base). 2008. *Responder knowledge base.* https://www.rkb.us (accessed March 19, 2008).

Steelnack, J. 2007. *OSHA Directorate of Standards and Compliance.* Presentation at the IOM Workshop, December 17, 2007, Washington, DC.

4

Emerging Issues and Research Areas in Personal Protective Technology

Given the relevance and substantive impact of the National Institute for Occupational Safety and Health (NIOSH) Personal Protective Technology Program,[1] (PPT Program) the committee provides this chapter as a forward look toward ensuring that the program is on the forefront of personal protective technologies. A full evaluation of emerging areas for PPT research and standards setting would require a comprehensive review of the field. This type of in-depth effort was not possible within the time allotted to the committee and the scope of its evaluation.

In this chapter, in keeping with the guidance from the Framework Document, the committee provides suggestions on future directions in materials technology, human factors, ensemble integration, safety culture, and training, as well as ideas relevant to emerging areas in several other technical areas that reflect the expertise of individual committee members. The committee has not conducted a formal assessment of needs in the field of PPT research.

PPT PROGRAM'S PROCESS FOR IDENTIFYING EMERGING ISSUES

An essential characteristic of a high-performing program is its ability to anticipate, identify, and respond to emerging needs or opportunities, including those

---

[1] As defined in Chapter 1, this report uses the term *PPT Program* to refer to the efforts from 2001 to the present that have been conducted by NIOSH relevant to the 12 PPT-relevant objectives that focus primarily on protection against respiratory and dermal hazards (Box 1-1).

caused by external factors outside the control of the program. The PPT Program has demonstrated in the case of standards setting for CBRN respirators that given the resources and the mandate, it can move rapidly and effectively to address highly complex needs.

In the evidence package provided to the committee and in subsequent discussions with NIOSH staff, the committee learned about the process by which the PPT Program's research priorities are determined and decisions are made about participation in standards-setting efforts. For the certification process, NIOSH is bound by federal mandate to perform respirator certification as specifically laid out in the Code of Federal Regulations. NIOSH, through the PPT Program, can and does take the initiative to update the certification requirements to adapt to new technologies; however, this continues to be a lengthy endeavor and increased efforts are needed to expedite revisions to the regulations (see Chapter 2). Further, increased website information on the progress of each modification in the federal rule-making process would help open the process and make it more transparent.

The PPT Program sets its research and other institutional priorities through an ongoing strategic planning process that culminates in an annual planning summit attended by the governance team comprised of key PPT Program managers. The governance team also meets periodically throughout the year to provide input into major decisions about emerging issues. The goals of the summit meeting are to conduct program assessments, identify priorities, and formulate the PPT Program budget for the coming year. This process began in 2006 as a National Personal Protective Technology Laboratory (NPPTL) planning summit and expanded in 2008 to include input from the broader PPT Program. The committee urges continued efforts in future planning to systematically consider the range of research gaps relevant to the many types of protective equipment and technologies.

As part of its strategic planning process, the PPT Program places an emphasis on obtaining input via stakeholder meetings held throughout the year with manufacturers, workers, researchers, regulatory personnel, and others (see Box 2-1). Most recently, the PPT Program held a public stakeholder meeting on March 6, 2008. The PPT Program has been the sole or joint sponsor of a number of PPT-related conferences, such as the 2005 conference *Advanced Personal Protective Equipment: Challenges in Protecting First Responders*. These conferences highlight new research and products and are an important input into development efforts. Results of intramural and extramural research also provide input to the process as do feedback and interactions with the many collaborating partner organizations and agencies.

On its website, NIOSH identifies the following emerging issues as top priorities for the PPT Program's efforts to provide effective NIOSH-certified respiratory protection equipment for all workers: CBRN protections, pandemic influenza preparedness, mine-related research, and nanotechnology (NIOSH, 2007).

In 2005, the PPT Program contracted with the Institute of Medicine (IOM) to establish a standing committee (the Committee on Personal Protective Equipment for Workplace Safety and Health) to provide ongoing discussions regarding strategic issues relevant to PPT. Additionally, the PPT Program has sponsored several IOM and National Research Council (NRC) studies that have examined specific issues (anthropometric research, planning for pandemic influenza, and surveillance) identified by the standing committee and by NIOSH staff (IOM, 2007, 2008; NRC, 2007). Recommendations from the resulting reports have been used by the PPT Program as a basis for research planning.

External factors can also drive the identification of new research issues or areas of focus (see Chapter 3). The 2001 terrorist attacks and the resulting national efforts to improve emergency response capabilities resulted in a number of PPT-related projects and efforts focused on improving the PPT for emergency responders. The threat of pandemic influenza and the 2003 outbreaks of severe acute respiratory syndrome (SARS) have also heightened interest in PPT for healthcare workers and for the general public.

COMMITTEE'S ASSESSMENT OF THE PPT PROGRAM'S PROCESS

The committee recognizes the many inputs to the PPT Program's process for establishing research priorities. The PPT Program has had a number of public meetings and is now engaged in focusing these meetings on the broader range of protective technologies. The PPT Program has been very successful in engaging specific and familiar stakeholder groups, including respirator manufacturers and the emergency response community, and recognizes the need to expand into other work sectors. Further, the PPT Program has demonstrated its engagement in PPT policy development through participation in consensus standards development committees and through its interactions with other federal agencies.

In developing its research priorities and other critical aspects of its program, the PPT Program needs to more closely follow a life-cycle approach to PPT testing with particular attention to increasing pre- and post-marketing field studies. This life-cycle approach should be implemented for all types of personal protective technologies. With regard to respirators, the development of standards establishes the basis for the certification program, which in turn would be supported by a series of pre-market and feasibility studies. Once fielded, the respirator equipment that has been certified is subject to product audits and manufacturing site audits. Additional field studies and more data from surveillance studies (discussed below) would be fundamental to implementing a truly iterative and cyclical process that yields ever-improved PPT.

The PPT Program's process for identifying and addressing emerging areas seems quite open and transparent, and the committee urges the PPT Program to continue in this manner as it reaches out to other workplace sectors. The PPT Program would also benefit from further expertise in behavioral sciences and interdisciplinary specialties, aimed principally at human factors. Given the ongoing challenges of workers' noncompliance with PPT use, it is paramount that NIOSH recognize psychosocial, usability, comfort, and behavioral issues that profoundly modify the relationship between PPT design and user compliance. As discussed later in the chapter, the committee believes that one of the critical issues for PPT is the integration of protective products into usable ensembles that are coupled and interface with each other without introducing new hazards or reducing the effectiveness of any single product within an ensemble.

In the committee's assessment, efforts are needed to more fully integrate the PPT Program into the matrix of the NIOSH organization. Only recently have efforts been made to integrate a PPT emphasis into some of the cross-cutting components of NIOSH such as the Health Hazard Evaluation (HHE) program and surveillance efforts. The PPT surveillance action plan (NIOSH, 2008e), for example, is a start in the right direction in that it assesses the capacity of ongoing and proposed surveillance activities across NIOSH to inform PPT research needs.

EMERGING ISSUES IDENTIFIED BY THE COMMITTEE

The committee identified several overarching emerging issues that affect all types of PPT. In addition, several specific areas for future research are suggested.

New Materials Technologies

Because the effectiveness of most PPT is dependent on acting as a barrier to hazardous agents, the usefulness of PPT can be jeopardized by ill-fitting, burdensome, or hard-to-wear products. This is especially a concern for respirators where even the most effective filter is only as good as the users' desire to don the respirator, the lack of leakage of the respirator, and the surety of fit. New materials technologies offer many opportunities for improving fit and comfort. A recent IOM report on personal protective equipment for healthcare workers (IOM, 2008) discussed some of the technologies on the near horizon including shape memory polymers. Further, rapidly evolving knowledge in materials sciences and engineering may yield as-yet-undefined technologies that could change the fundamental nature of PPT and perhaps eventually develop protective mechanisms that negate the need for PPT.

The PPT Program plans to hold a workshop in late 2008 to examine the technologies available to move toward a "fits-all" or "universal-fit" respirator that could

EMERGING ISSUES AND RESEARCH AREAS

easily and effectively conform to all face types and would not require fit testing. The committee believes that workshops such as this one are an excellent example of the PPT Program's leadership in this area and encourages NIOSH to continue to explore cutting-edge technologies by bringing together experts of diverse design, engineering, technological, and behavioral backgrounds.

Usability and Human Factors

One of the major weaknesses of PPT is its dependence on the individual user. PPT can protect only when worn as designed—a simple fact, but one that has many ramifications: workers need to see the value of wearing PPT; they must use the equipment correctly in order to be protected against the hazard; they have to be able to accomplish their work tasks while wearing the equipment; and they need to be comfortable while wearing PPT so that they will continue to wear it.

PPT development and application pose two significant challenges. The first is to ensure that the equipment is efficacious, providing protection from the hazard for which it is designed. The second is effectiveness so that when used in the workplace, PPT provides the intended protection, fits a variety of human shapes in a highly diverse workforce, and is user-friendly. A growing realization is that comfort is a safety issue. Other key aspects of usability are durability and serviceability since there must be a high confidence that PPT will continue to provide adequate protection for the duration of the planned tasks under foreseeable conditions. Designing for usability spans several disciplines including engineering, behavioral sciences, training systems design, and human resources management, as well as interdisciplinary specialties such as human factors. The extent to which PPT can be designed to be efficacious, usable, practical, and effective in the context of its use will rest on the extent to which the PPT Program integrates different disciplines into the design, development, and evaluation of PPT. For example, the burden on miners of using a self-contained self-rescuer (SCSR) in an emergency escape needs to be evaluated and considered on an integrated basis. This evaluation should address the use of an SCSR in the context of high temperature, high humidity, and high metabolic rate.

Systematic laboratory- and field-based studies need to be conducted that support the development of performance goals and technologies for heat stress reduction and other physiologic burdens resulting from wearing PPT. The impact of protective equipment on the susceptibility of users to heat stroke is an important area of inquiry. The PPT Program has recently added a physiology laboratory and now has the capacity to expand its work in this discipline. The committee urges increased efforts in this important area.

The value of addressing design and usability is only beginning to be fully recognized in PPT and related areas, although it has been an important feature of product design and evaluation in many other industries. Considerable progress has been made in adapting laboratory procedures to improve fit, but much more work remains to be done to address gender differences and the wide variation of sizes, shapes, and heights across an increasingly diverse worker population. Poor fit of protective equipment and clothing is a serious issue for men with small- or large-size frames and for many women workers. Indeed, much of the technology of PPT has evolved without consideration of the variations in frames and features; work needs to be done to enhance gender equity in PPT design. The significant growth of the number of females in nontraditional workplaces, such as the construction trades, lends some urgency to the need for attention to issues of fit and usability.

Some initial work designed to improve awareness and research on issues concerning women and the use of personal protective equipment has been the result of a NIOSH-Department of Labor (DoL) working group on women and PPT. The working group has commissioned the design of a survey to obtain data on the PPT needs of women; the PPT equipment they wear; and their views on the comfort, fit, and usability of that equipment (American Society of Safety Engineers, 2007). Initial cognitive assessments have been undertaken with a pilot cohort of 21 women and men of short stature in construction, mining, law enforcement, and health care (MSHA, 2007). The committee encourages the NIOSH PPT Program to become further involved in these efforts and to expand work to improve PPT for individuals across a broad spectrum of body frames and features.

Although much work has been done on developing consensus standards for the performance effectiveness of PPT (particularly as related to respirators), few standards exist regarding wearability and physiologic burden. The PPT Program, along with manufacturers, employers, workers, and standards development organizations, needs to work toward setting such standards.

PPT Ensembles and Systems Integration

Many hazardous workplace situations require workers to use multiple types of PPT. Firefighters face the respiratory hazards of smoke inhalation while at the same time confronting the challenges of extreme heat and flames that pose dangers to all parts of the body. Healthcare workers concerned with exposure to bloodborne pathogens need protection for all potential exposure points including the eyes, mouth, nose, and broken skin. Construction workers may need protection from the noise of their equipment while also requiring respiratory protection from dust and the safety of fall protection technologies for jobs at dangerous heights.

Seamless integration of various types of PPT is thus critically important. PPT ensembles bring to mind coats and gloves and helmets but also should include a range of products that allow multiple protective technologies to be added without gaps or loss of protection (for example, respirators need to integrate with both eye protection and hearing protection). Similarly, workers must be shielded from hazardous atmospheres without impeding seeing, hearing, and communication. Developing PPT ensembles will need to involve the standardization of fittings and seals so that PPT components and technologies can be truly integrated and interoperable. PPT Program staff members have worked with the International Association of Fire Fighters and others to develop and test ensembles for firefighters that integrate protective and functional gloves into firefighter coats.

A focus is needed on innovations that can provide workers and employers with protective ensembles and interfaces appropriate for the varying PPT needs across different occupations and industries. Input from the National Occupational Research Agenda (NORA) Sector Councils and extramural partners can be useful in focusing on the relevant PPT issues.

Advancements in PPT may also have to be considered in the design of environmental controls. For example, a new comprehensive program should be considered that takes a fresh look at all of the hazards that miners face in carrying out their jobs in both underground and surface mining. A complete PPT ensemble approach should incorporate all of the PPT needed to address all identified hazards. The specific hazards addressed should consider routine exposures such as noise, heat, particulate inhalation from diesel and coal dust, and ergonomic challenges, as well as the emergency hazards for which mine escape respirators (SCSRs) were designed. SCSRs are intended to provide miners with a temporary supply of air for safe escape from roof falls, fires, and other emergencies in underground mines. Advances in communications and individual miner location technology, which are also relevant to firefighters and emergency responders, should be considered.

Additional efforts will be necessary to develop effective test methods and performance criteria for PPT ensembles. Standardization is needed for the interface between PPT components, so that, for example, eye protection from one manufacturer is compatible with respirators from another manufacturer.

Establishing or Enhancing Workplace Safety Culture

Workplaces vary widely in the extent to which worker safety is an innate and valued part of the work culture. Although most U.S. employers are required to follow Occupational Safety and Health Administration (OSHA) regulations on workplace safety and mining employers are required to follow Mine Safety and Health Administration (MSHA) requirements, there are few guidelines to assist employers with metrics or indicators to conduct quantitative and qualitative analyses of the safety culture and its impact on the use of PPT. From the employer to the supervisor to the worker, a workplace culture that values safety—and consequently a workplace climate that reinforces the safety culture—provides an environment of cooperation and compliance that supports the establishment of effective administrative controls and proactive safety programs.

Although the PPT Program is focused on only one aspect of the workplace safety issue, it is important that NIOSH emphasize systems safety approaches that support the importance of improving all components of workplace safety in order to ensure that each individual PPT component is optimized. The increase in the percentage of contingent and self-employed workers in the workforce presents a significant safety culture challenge. These workers may not be covered by OSHA regulations and may lack training in the selection and wear of PPT equipment. Further research is needed on improving the workplace culture of safety across industries and occupations, and the PPT Program should play a significant leadership role in conducting research on how to increase worker adherence to using PPT as a part of its broader efforts.

Training and Professional Education

The PPT Program's respirator certification process results in a wide variety of high-quality, commercially available, NIOSH-certified respirators. Additionally, the PPT Program is playing a growing role in ensuring the development of high standards for efficacy of other types of PPT (e.g., gloves). However, the level of protection that this equipment provides the end user depends on how (and whether) it is used and maintained. The level of training, the motivation, and the actions of the end user will determine whether the equipment is being used at all, whether it is used properly, and whether the user is provided with appropriate protection. OSHA regulatory requirements mandate that work sites using respirators provide a respirator training program; best practices in those programs need to be identified and disseminated. An assessment of current training and fit testing programs and respirator use should be carried out by the PPT Program, in collaboration with its many partners, to identify pressing training and educational issues and to develop the materials and programs essential to meet those needs. Efforts are also needed to improve recognition and response to the NIOSH certification seal and to evaluate and improve package inserts and accompanying instructions for all types of PPT. NIOSH is one of many responsible agencies and organizations that can and should provide its substantive expertise in addressing training issues.

In 2006, the PPT Program asked the NIOSH Education and Research Centers (ERCs) for information on the extent to which PPT-related topics are incorporated into ERC curricula and professional training. The responses showed some limited efforts in this area but pointed to a substantial need for improved education and professional training on the role of PPT in occupational safety and health.

The NIOSH PPT Program should work with OSHA, MSHA, manufacturers, professional associations, and other relevant partners to identify training materials needed by employers, employees, and purchasers of all types of PPT. Training materials developed as a result of that effort should be available in multiple formats and languages. The PPT Program should increase its collaboration with the NIOSH ERCs to integrate the relevant features of PPT into ongoing training and education efforts.

Additional Emerging Issues

The committee identified a number of specific issues that it sees as new or expanding areas of research. This is not meant to be an exhaustive list but rather a brief synopsis of some emerging research, standards-setting, and certification challenges.

Incorporating Sensor, Telemetry, and Communications Technologies

PPT such as SCSRs and firefighter ensembles are often used in emergency or rescue situations, and it is critical to incorporate relevant sensors and systems into this equipment that will allow individual workers to be tracked and aided in escape or will allow others to find them. For example, a detection or telemetry system could be added to an SCSR respirator to identify the time and location at which a miner has begun to use the equipment and any other information that would lead to a more rapid rescue. Usage sensors, indicating the amount of oxygen used, could be developed for SCSRs along with improved sensors for end-of-service-life indicators.

The use of PPT equipment often constrains communication between workers. For example, respirators limit the clarity and strength of verbal communication. Thus, advances in communication technologies should also be considered an integral part of the PPT research program. Although these technologies often go beyond the purview of traditional PPT, the committee urges the PPT Program to continue to provide innovative leadership in facilitating partnerships that can assess the entire work environment to identify opportunities for improving the utility of PPT for worker safety within a context that integrates these other important factors, such as communication devices and rescue protocols.

Chemical Protective Clothing

The needs for research in the area of protection against dermal exposure to hazardous agents have been known for quite a while, but resources have limited progress to date. As discussed in Chapter 2, much less is known about occupational limits for dermal exposures in comparison with the large body of knowledge and detailed exposure limits for respiratory hazards. It is therefore difficult to select the appropriate dermal protective products and to assess their effectiveness in the workplace. As discussed in earlier chapters, NIOSH (through the PPT Program and the Dermal Exposure Research Program) is involved in research efforts to address some of these concerns. The committee hopes that resources can be found to address and prioritize research needs for improvements in protective clothing that will reduce exposure to dermal hazards.

Filter Media

The composition of filter media for respirators has evolved into a complex blend of fibers of various sizes, which in some cases is enhanced with an electrostatic charge to provide the desired filter efficiency. The electrostatic charge on some filter fibers can be dissipated by environmental conditions such as temperature and humidity as well as by organic solvents and oils. The PPT Program has recognized the need to examine the effect of workplace conditions such as organic vapor exposure on electrostatic filter performance. A program partnership with North Carolina State University has resulted in a series of articles evaluating the effect of organic chemical exposure on the performance of electrostatic and mechanical fibers and filter media (Jasper et al., 2006; Kim et al., 2006). Further research is needed to develop a more detailed technical understanding of the properties of electrostatic charge on filter media and how it can be dissipated under workplace conditions. Currently filters are tested by NIOSH and certified, but no description of the filter medium is required as part of the certification process. However, filter composition and technology are important in determining how frequently filters need to be replaced. The PPT Program should consider requiring as part of the certification process the respirator manufacturer to provide a description of the filter medium and its limitations, particularly the conditions under which the filtration performance or the filter material itself may degrade. The information should also be made available to purchasers and end users to aid in the selection of respirators and to develop filter change-out schedules.

Flow Rates

The selection of proper flow rates for testing respirator equipment is important to worker protection. Flow rate tests are used to simulate the breathing of workers at different work rates in different environments. In devising these tests, there are important trade-offs to be kept in mind. The rates must be high enough to ensure that the equipment provides adequate protection but not so high that they become an unnecessary physiologic burden for the user or an unnecessary work hindrance. For example, to attain high flow rates for powered air-purifying respirators (PAPRs), manufacturers currently rely on a relatively large motor and blower, which, for some occupations such as health care, can seriously interfere with worker communication and mobility.

Currently, chemical warfare agent tests for air-purifying respirators, PAPRs, and escape respirators use flow rates of 40 liters per minute (42 CFR 84), as does the flow rate test used to certify self-contained breathing apparatus (SCBA). The National Fire Protection Association (NFPA) standard for SCBAs (NFPA, 2007) required a breathing machine flow rate of 100 liters per minute; this value was identified as the breathing rate of a firefighter working at or near capacity (Burgess, 1976). Increases in the respiratory demand flow rate during intense physical activity need to be further studied particularly regarding their implications for respirators and other forms of PPT (Kaufman and Hastings, 2005).

Further research is needed to develop a set of flow rates appropriate to the type of respirator and sensitive to the intended use and physiological demands of potential users. Test protocols that reflect the array of work environments would allow respirator manufacturers to use different design criteria and potentially more efficient filter media.

Hazard and Control Framework

Employers need to be able to decide what types of controls are needed based on the risks faced by workers. Developing a framework in which to view the relationship between exposures and hazards is a recognized need in occupational health that has implications for PPT selection and use. The linkage between hazard and control was explicitly made in the National Occupational Hazard Survey (1972-1974) but has not been the subject of recent surveillance activity. Although this work is relevant throughout NIOSH it is important that the PPT Program be involved to ensure that PPT is considered in this effort.

One methodology is suggested by "control banding," a technique that is detailed in a model by the Health and Safety Executive in the United Kingdom (HSE, 2008). Control banding categorizes the type of controls needed to prevent hazardous occupational exposures. The control banding process identifies a single control technology (e.g., general ventilation) that is applicable to a range or band of exposure levels to a chemical (e.g., 1 to 10 mg/m^3) and that falls within a given hazard group (e.g., skin and eye irritants). Four main control bands have been developed for exposure to chemicals by inhalation (NIOSH, 2008b):

- Band 1: Use good industrial hygiene practice and general ventilation.
- Band 2: Use local exhaust ventilation.
- Band 3: Enclose the process.
- Band 4: Seek expert advice.

A framework or guideline for employers and employees would be a significant starting point for informed decision making about environmental, administrative, and PPT controls.

Anthropometrics

The committee hopes that in the long term, the need for respirator fit testing will be made obsolete by technological breakthroughs in environmental, engineering, or administrative controls or in materials that conform easily to the shape of a variety of faces. However, specific smart technologies may be in the distant future, and there is currently a strong need to further the knowledge base on the anthropometric variability of the worker population. Collaboration with other research and practice organizations focused on smart technologies and anthropometric variability is encouraged. The PPT Program sponsored an IOM study (IOM, 2007) specifically focused on these issues and has provided a detailed response to the IOM committee report (NIOSH, 2008c). Emerging areas discussed in that report include replacing the current use of isoamyl acetate with quantitative measures evaluating user seal check, utilizing the panel for certification of filtering facepiece respirators, modifications in the certification requirements to encourage manufacturers to develop sizes to fit underrepresented anthropometric categories, and improving the description of face mask sizes in manufacturer's literature.

Development of a clearly defined protocol and sampling frame for three-dimensional imaging is needed. Because of the highly specialized equipment required to conduct anthropometric research, the committee urges the PPT Program to establish cooperative agreements with centers capable of performing three-dimensional imaging. Furthermore, it will be important to develop a central web-based repository for these data that is accessible and easy to use by the research and practice community.

Pandemic Influenza

In response to the potential for an influenza pandemic and in light of the important role that PPT played in the SARS outbreaks, the PPT Program has begun research to address relevant issues such as mechanisms for decontamination of PPT. Many other important research questions remain. The PPT Program through input from the IOM Committee on Personal Protective Equipment for Workplace Safety and Health requested an IOM study focused on PPT for healthcare workers in the event of pandemic influenza that addressed many of the research needs outlined below (IOM, 2008). The PPT Program has recently released an action plan in response to that report (NIOSH, 2008d).

Because of the many unknowns regarding transmission of influenza, the committee urges NIOSH and other agencies in the Centers for Disease Control and Prevention (CDC) to expedite research to address a range of short- and long-term needs including the following:

- Assessing the viability of virus particles on nondisposable and disposable respirators and other PPT
- Developing effective decontamination methods—this is particularly critical for healthcare workers who interact with many patients and staff members over the course of a day
- Understanding the hazards posed by viral particle size and aerosolization from a human cough and the impact on the design of PPT
- Assessing physiological factors that favor or fail to support N95 use when covered by a surgical mask

Nanotechnology

Much remains to be learned about the extent to which nanoparticles pose a health hazard. This is an area where NIOSH has moved out ahead of the curve to examine occupational health concerns.

The committee did not fully examine the many emerging issues relevant to nanotechnology but urges the PPT Program to continue to keep abreast of efforts in this field and to continue to assess the efficacy of filters and respirators in protecting against exposures to ever-smaller particles. In addition, the PPT Program is encouraged to ensure that the aforementioned considerations such as human factors and other understudied determinants of effectiveness are taken into account.

Surveillance

The PPT Program is in the midst of decisions regarding future surveillance activities and a draft PPT surveillance action plan has recently been released (NIOSH, 2008e). Several options for prospective surveillance efforts that may yield focused and useful information come with a fairly significant price tag and would require a long time horizon for data collection and analysis. However, in the judgment of the committee, the protection against survey error and survey bias that only a prospective cohort methodology can provide is likely to be well worth the investment of time, money, and personnel required to obtain such data. Other options under consideration include incorporating PPT data collection into several ongoing surveys. Additional sources of information stemming from archival administrative records that currently exist should also be considered while awaiting the anticipated data from long-term prospective surveillance.

The NIOSH Health Hazard Evaluation Program[2] could be a valuable source of data to inform the PPT Program. Under the HHE Program, NIOSH provides assistance to employers or employees in determining whether chemical, physical, biological, or other agents are hazardous as used or found in the workplace. More than 8,000 evaluations have been completed since the inception of the HHE Program in 1972. According to the program's database, more than 1,000 reports have addressed respiratory hazards and some 640 have addressed dermal hazards (NIOSH, 2008a). These technical reports have often described PPT practices directly observed in the workplace and have made recommendations for appropriate PPT to address the hazards associated with specific exposures. PPT Program staff members have stated that collaborative efforts with the HHE Program are underway. The committee finds value in increased use of this potential resource for improving PPT use in the workplace. The program should focus on developing systematic secondary data analysis methods and working out protocols and frameworks to collect and extract relevant information that can be used in the evaluation and design of PPT.

Information from the HHE Program and other sources can eventually be used in the National Occupational Exposure Database, currently under development by NIOSH (NIOSH, 2002). This central repository of occupational exposure-related information will initially hold newly acquired and legacy exposure-related data generated by NIOSH in addition to exposure data from sources outside NIOSH. The database will document, for each sample collected, process and task descriptions, engineering controls, PPT in use, and information on analytical methods. In addition, it will contain descriptors of the study facilities, agents, standardized industry and occupational codes, ergonomics, and work organization. The goal is a system that would eventually include end outcome data and would provide valuable surveillance-generated information to inform the PPT Program and other occupational health efforts.

REFERENCES

American Society of Safety Engineers. 2007. *Tales from the front: NIOSH/DoL Working Group on Women and PPE*. http://www.asse.org/professionalaffairs/govtaffairs/gaupdate/index.php?issue=2007-11-13&article=719 (accessed May 20, 2008).

---

[2] The HHE Program is the subject of a separate National Academies' evaluation.

Burgess, W. H. 1976. *Design specifications for respiratory breathing devises for firefighters.* Department of Health, Education and Welfare Publication No. 76-121.

HSE (Health and Safety Executive). 2008. *Easy steps to control health risks from chemicals.* http://www.coshh-essentials.org.uk (accessed March 18, 2008).

IOM (Institute of Medicine). 2007. *Assessment of the NIOSH head-and-face anthropometric survey of U.S. respirator users.* Washington, DC: The National Academies Press.

IOM. 2008. *Preparing for an influenza pandemic: Personal protective equipment for healthcare workers.* Washington, DC: The National Academies Press.

Jasper, W., J. Hinestroza, A. Mohan, J. Kim, B. Shiels, M. Gunay, D. Thompson, and R. Barker. 2006. Effect of xylene exposure on the performance of electret filter media. *Journal of Aerosol Science* 47(7):903-911.

Kaufman, J. W., and S. Hastings. 2005. Respiratory demand during rigorous physical work in a chemical protective ensemble. *Journal of Occupational and Environmental Hygiene* 2:98-110.

Kim, J., W. Jasper, and J. Hinestroza. 2006. Charge characterization of an electrically charged fiber via electrostatic force microscopy. *Journal of Engineered Fibers and Fabrics* 1(2):30-46.

MSHA (Mine Safety and Health Administration). 2007. *Presentation by Laura McMullen, MSHA to the IOM Committee,* December 17, 2007.

NFPA (National Fire Protection Association). 2007. *NFPA 1981: Standard on open-circuit self-contained breathing apparatus (SCBA) for emergency services,* 2007 edition.

NIOSH (National Institute for Occupational Safety and Health). 2002. *Exposure assessment methods: Research needs and priorities.* NIOSH Publication Number 2002-126. http://www.cdc.gov/niosh/docs/2002-126/2002-126.html#Data%20Collection (accessed April 24, 2008).

NIOSH. 2007. *NIOSH program portfolio, personal protective technology. Emerging issues.* http://www.cdc.gov/niosh/programs/ppt/emerging.html (accessed April 8, 2008).

NIOSH. 2008a. *Health hazard evaluations.* http://www.cdc.gov/niosh/hhe/ (accessed April 8, 2008).

NIOSH. 2008b. *Control banding.* http://www.cdc.gov/niosh/topics/ctrlbanding/ (accessed April 24, 2008).

NIOSH. 2008c. *NPPTL facial anthropometrics research roadmap.* http://www.cdc.gov/niosh/review/public/111/ (accessed March 4, 2008).

NIOSH. 2008d. *Personal protective equipment (PPE) for healthcare workers action plan.* http://www.cdc.gov/niosh/review/public/129/ (accessed March 5, 2008).

NIOSH. 2008e. *PPT surveillance program action plan. Draft, March 5, 2008* (accessible through the National Academies Public Access File).

NRC (National Research Council). 2007. *Measuring respirator use in the workplace.* Washington, DC: The National Academies Press.

5

Recommendations for PPT Program Improvement

Millions of working Americans depend on personal protective technologies (PPT) to prevent exposures to occupational health hazards. As described in the preceding chapters, the committee believes that the NIOSH PPT Program has effectively identified and implemented high-priority research and standards-setting efforts and has been thorough and forward thinking in conducting the respirator certification process. Further, the committee finds that the PPT Program has made a substantive impact on improving worker safety and health by ensuring that NIOSH-certified respirators meet rigorous pre-specified criteria and by the formation of strong partnerships with other organizations and agencies working to develop rigorous PPT standards. The NIOSH PPT Program has made effective use of its limited resources and has moved the research, standards-setting, and certification agendas forward, largely with a focus on respirators. However, much still has not been done due to serious budgetary constraints. The committee offers the following recommendations with the goal of improving the ability of the NIOSH PPT Program to broaden its scope and depth of responsibility in order to protect workers more effectively from hazardous workplace exposures, illness, injuries, and disease.

IMPLEMENT AND SUSTAIN A COMPREHENSIVE NATIONAL PPT PROGRAM

Recommendation 1: Implement and Sustain a Comprehensive National Personal Protective Technology Program

NIOSH should work to ensure the implementation of the 2001 congressional mandate for a comprehensive state-of-the-art federal program focused on personal protective technology. A comprehensive program would build on the current NIOSH PPT Program and would bring unified responsibility and oversight to all PPT-related activity at NIOSH. The National Personal Protective Technology Program should

- Oversee, coordinate, and where appropriate, conduct research across all types of occupational PPT and across all relevant occupations and workplaces;
- Participate in policy development and standards setting across all types of occupational PPT;
- Oversee all PPT certification in order to ensure a minimum uniform standard of protection and wearability. The National Program should collaborate with other relevant government agencies, private-sector organizations, and not-for-profit organizations to conduct an assessment of the certification mechanisms needed to ensure the efficacy of all types of PPT; and
- Promote the development, standards setting, and certification of effectively integrated PPT components and ensembles in which multiple types of PPT (e.g., eye protection, hearing protection, respirators) can be effectively and seamlessly worn together.

The committee was struck by the discordance between the congressional mandate[1] to establish the National Personal Protective Technology Laboratory

---

[1] Senate Report 106-293 stated "It has been brought to the Committee's attention the need for design, testing and state-of-the-art equipment for this nation's 50 million miners, firefighters, healthcare, agricultural and industrial workers.... The Committee encourages NIOSH to carry out research, testing and related activities aimed at protecting workers, who respond to public health needs in the event of a terrorist incident. The Committee encourages CDC [the Centers for Disease Control and Prevention] to organize and implement a national personal protective equipment laboratory."

(NPPTL) in 2001 and the challenges faced by the current PPT Program, which focuses almost solely on respiratory PPT because of limited resources. If NIOSH is to respond fully to its 2001 congressional directive to develop and test state-of-the-art national PPT needs (respirators, protective clothing, gloves, hearing protection, eye protection, and other types of PPT) across all relevant work sectors, then a more comprehensive approach is needed. The National PPT Program should be responsible for all PPT efforts within NIOSH, as well as for coordinating relevant efforts with federal agencies (Department of Defense [DoD], Department of Homeland Security [DHS], Food and Drug Administration [FDA], Department of Labor [DoL], and Environmental Protection Agency [EPA]).

The designation of the National Personal Protective Technology Laboratory as a *laboratory*, denotes the important function of research, but does not fully capture the scope of efforts that are needed to improve worker safety through personal protective technologies. Designating these efforts as the National PPT *Program* emphasizes the goal of coordinating and expanding the full range of certification, standards-setting, and research efforts.

As PPT becomes increasingly complex, integration of its many components requires scrupulously coordinated development of interfaces and ensembles that are designed, standardized, and certified under the oversight of a single entity within NIOSH, dedicated solely to PPT in the workplace. To promote worker safety by integrating various types of protective equipment requires placing the responsibility for all PPT efforts at NIOSH under a single entity that has the responsibility and the requisite resources to oversee the broad array of PPT and to lead the efforts to provide workers with improved and innovative protective equipment. Further, the consolidation of PPT responsibilities and the focus on the wide array of PPT devices could be leveraged to expand recall authority for defective products (e.g., older models of PASS [personal alert safety system] warning devices). The National PPT Program should examine PPT interface issues and should work with relevant partners to coordinate and oversee the research, certification, and standards setting for all PPT, including multicomponent ensembles.

In 2005, NIOSH took a significant first step toward coordinating PPT-related efforts across the institute by establishing the PPT Program and developing a matrix approach to management. However, the committee is concerned that the current matrix structure of PPT efforts at NIOSH may be too ambiguously configured to serve the long-term needs and flexible goals of a comprehensive, coordinated national PPT endeavor. Although designated as a program in name, the directors of the current PPT Program have limited budgetary authority and management responsibility for PPT research and other efforts outside NPPTL. As a result of the lack of a single authority, there are major gaps in the integration, coordination, and consolidation of many types of PPT. The current matrix approach, while a good first step, does not bring the full depth and range of NIOSH expertise to bear on moving forward in improving and coordinating PPT at the national level. In examining the PPT needs of one specific workplace sector, a recent Institute of Medicine committee examined the anticipated PPT needs of healthcare workers during an influenza pandemic and recommended that Congress expand the resources provided to NIOSH for expediting the development and approval of improved PPT (IOM, 2008). The National PPT Program, through a much broader focus, proportionately increased responsibilities, and more direct lines of coordinated oversight and responsibility would provide the needed impetus for an integrated approach to PPT that encompasses the entire range of protective equipment and technologies and the multiple interfaces between and among them.

After evaluating the evidence and hearing from many stakeholders, the committee has concluded that NIOSH certification of respirators (through its extensive testing and audit process) has had a significant positive impact on the quality of respirators available in the workplace. However, there is no analogous federal process for ensuring the certification of non-respiratory PPT (e.g., eye protection, hearing protection, protective clothing). Currently, third-party certification is an available voluntary option for several specific types of protective clothing, gloves, and helmets, but there is no uniform oversight of the certification process for all PPT. Other types of protective equipment (e.g., protective eyewear, protective footwear) are often manufactured to meet performance criteria specified by consensus standards, which are voluntary. The committee is therefore concerned about the lack of rigorous certification for some types of PPT and encourages a thorough assessment of certification and oversight options. There are several possible ways in which an expanded PPT Program might bring a minimum standard of uniformity to the safety of workers who are dependent on PPT: (1) The PPT Program could be designated with certification responsibilities as is currently done with respirators. (2) An alternative option would be to provide the National PPT Program with oversight authority to ensure that PPT products meet uniform consensus standards. The program's oversight role could include providing support to identify and resolve any procedural or technical issues or conflicts that may arise in the course of certification of personal protective equipment by federally licensed private-sector laboratories. (3) Establishing a set of NIOSH-approved independent testing laboratories is yet another option, such as is done for the testing of bulletproof vests by National Institute of Justice-approved laboratories. The committee did not have the mandate to examine these or other options thoroughly but urges a detailed assessment of these issues with the goal of developing and implementing a standardized process to certify all types of PPT.

The PPT Program has utilized its own laboratory effectively and has nurtured a number of partnerships. These collaborative efforts, particularly as seen in the work on CBRN respirators, have fostered positive results. Increased collaborations across NIOSH divisions and sectors are needed, as well as efforts to collaborate with additional federal, nonprofit, and for-profit agencies and organizations. The committee urges the PPT Program to continue to assert its role as a resource and to expand its leadership role in initiating dialogue about critical PPT issues and exploring new and innovative technologies.

The committee believes that a meaningfully integrated approach to improving all types of occupational PPT would logically require consolidation of the oversight responsibilities for PPT efforts at NIOSH. The committee's emphasis in response to its charge was on proposing a general strategy intended to optimize the wealth of relevant expertise at NIOSH in order to meet the new challenges of developing fully integrated and coordinated protective ensembles and technologies for worker protection. Approaches could range from maintaining current laboratory and research facilities with changes in reporting and budgetary authority to more major organizational changes. Carrying out the original congressional intent of an effort focused on "the design, testing, and state-of-the-art [personal protective] equipment for this nation's . . . workers" (Senate Report 106-293) will necessitate a commitment to a broad scope of work and collaborative efforts that will impact workers in all occupations that use personal protective technologies.

ESTABLISH PPT RESEARCH CENTERS OF EXCELLENCE

Recommendation 2: Establish PPT Research Centers of Excellence and Increase Extramural PPT Research

The PPT Program should establish and sustain extramural PPT centers of excellence and work to increase other extramural research opportunities. The PPT Program should

- Develop and support research centers of excellence that work closely with the NIOSH intramural research program to improve PPT, increase field research, and explore and implement research to practice interventions; and
- Work with the NIOSH Office of Extramural Programs to increase other research opportunities and enhance collaboration and awareness of relevant PPT research efforts among intramural and extramural researchers.

The community of extramural scientists is a highly valuable resource for improving PPT. It is critical that this breadth and depth of expertise is focused on important PPT research questions relevant to improving PPT and to transferring PPT research into workplace practice. Successful efforts to address critical issues in many other fields of scientific inquiry have been the result of investing in extramural research centers of excellence. Research centers of excellence allow for interdisciplinary expertise and improved ability to evaluate interventions such as new technologies, while facilitating strong collaborations. Increased intramural research resources and personnel, extramural grants, cooperative agreements, and direct contracts should be balanced to leverage PPT capabilities. Where feasible, the PPT Program should take advantage of existing expertise, laboratory infrastructure, and outreach networks, which may be costly to duplicate in the intramural PPT Program. In addition to expanding the resources dedicated to PPT research and development, a strong extramural community provides the opportunity to extend scientific inquiry into the behavioral sciences and other types of expertise that might not be available within the NIOSH PPT Program. PPT centers of excellence should be aligned with one or more of the scientific focus areas of the PPT Program. The centers could be developed to be topic-specific (e.g., heat stress, dermal permeation) or to be sector-specific to explore the unique PPT needs of a particular occupation or set of workers. Several types of centers would be optimal. University-based research centers could establish collaborative networks with other universities and with nonprofit organizations and federal agencies focused on research and development of innovative approaches to PPT. Complementary centers of excellence would be those that are centered in nonprofit organizations, state departments of health or labor, or agencies with capabilities and expertise in post-market or field research. These centers, in conjunction with partner organizations and universities, could increase field research, and explore and implement research to practice interventions. Multi-year funding and evaluation are critical to build a strong and ever-improving research base.

Models of federally supported centers of excellence include those funded by the Department of Homeland Security, such as the National Center for the Study of Preparedness and Catastrophic Event Response, led by Johns Hopkins University (DHS, 2008) and the Nursing Centers of Excellence (funded by the National Institute of Nursing Research). Relevant examples of successful university-based centers of research in PPT include the University of Minnesota's Center for Filtration Research, North Carolina State University's Center for Research on Textile Protection and Comfort, and the University of Maryland's research focus on physiological testing. The National Construction Center, which is administered by The Center for Construction Research and Training, is an example of a national nonprofit consortium focused on research to practice.

Centers of excellence have advantages that come with developing a strong cadre of extramural investigators who can obtain research support and develop sustained careers in PPT—opportunities that are now largely nonexistent. Several committee members and workshop speakers noted this as a major impediment to choosing PPT research as a career path. Research support should be available for early career investigators to enable a viable career path for talented scientists.

The committee urges the PPT Program to sponsor an annual conference to facilitate interaction and exchange of ideas among intramural and extramural investigators working in PPT and relevant fields. The PPT Program's public stakeholder meetings, such as the one in March 2008, provide additional opportunity for researchers to discuss innovative research and identify new and emerging issues in PPT.

The PPT Program, through the NIOSH Office of Extramural Programs (OEP), has assembled a list of extramural grants relevant to PPT (Chapter 2). PPT Program staff members have also reported increased opportunities for dialogue with OEP in the past year regarding priorities for funding. The committee urges NIOSH to consider ways in which the PPT Program could have greater input into the extramural priority process at NIOSH and increased participation in drafting requests for grant applications. Further, the PPT Program and OEP should examine whether the current grant review structure (e.g., study groups) is adequately configured to review applications with expertise relevant to PPT.

Collaborative extramural partnerships, exemplified by centers of research excellence in personal protective technologies, would serve to leverage the PPT Program's resources and expertise and provide the coordinated intramural-extramural approach necessary for advancing science and technology relevant to protecting workers through PPT.

ENHANCE THE RESPIRATOR CERTIFICATION PROCESS

Recommendation 3: Enhance the Respirator Certification Process

The PPT Program should continue to improve the respirator certification process. The program should

- Expedite the revision of the respirator certification regulations. As a part of that effort, NIOSH should revise the respirator certification fee schedules so that certification fees paid by respirator manufacturers fully cover the cost of certification. NIOSH's research budget for PPT research should not be eroded by the costs of certification.
- Develop a mechanism for registering the purchase of NIOSH-certified respirators so that post-marketing notifications and recalls can be accomplished expeditiously and effectively.

- **Expand the audit programs to ensure that results of the product audit program are methodologically and statistically sound and that the site audit program ensures standardized quality of audits whether performed by NIOSH staff or contractors.**
- **Disseminate respirator certification test result data (e.g., breathing resistance).**

Respirator certification has been a significant part of the work of the PPT Program. In FY 2007, almost half (approximately 48 percent) of the PPT Program's $13.1 million budget was designated for the certification program (Table 2-2; data include overhead costs); in prior years, certification generally constituted about a third of the program's total budget. In FY 2007, certification occupied about half of the PPT Program's full-time equivalent workforce (Table 2-3). As highlighted in Chapters 2 and 3, the NIOSH respirator certification process is highly respected and provides a major contribution to worker safety. The committee believes that although the enhancements to the certification program recommended above will require additional resources, the dividends that will accrue to workers from improved standards, audits, and information dissemination will make such an investment sustainable and well worth the start-up costs.

Improving respirators, and thereby reducing exposures to respiratory hazards, is in large part an effort focused on updating, refining, and developing the tests and performance criteria that respirators must meet to provide effective protection in the workplace. These tests are specified through federal regulations, many of which have not been changed significantly in more than 35 years. The PPT Program through NPPTL has developed a modular approach to updating federal regulations. The committee sees these revisions and additions to the regulatory standards as a major opportunity for the PPT Program to improve respirators through updated tests that address current and evolving technologies. It is particularly important for current respirator workplace applications to be considered in the revision of respirator certification regulations. The proposed changes and additions to the regulations should be moved more expeditiously through the rule-making pipeline.

An issue of concern to the committee was the extent of federal resources devoted to the costs of respirator certification, costs that would more appropriately be borne by respirator manufacturers as is done for other types of product certification. The Bureau of Mines established the structure of certification fees in the approval schedule for each respirator type when each schedule was put in place. When the respirator certification program was transferred from the Bureau of Mines to the Mining Enforcement and Safety Administration (the predecessor of MSHA) and NIOSH in 1972, the fee structure from the previously existing Bureau of Mines approval schedules was incorporated into the new consolidated approval regulations without any change to the fees. Because the fee schedule has not been updated for over 35 years, the program covers only a small fraction of the current costs of respirator certification. Less than 10 percent of the cost of testing and certifying traditional respirators[2] is currently recovered through fees charged to manufacturers (see Chapter 2). Recent changes to the regulations have allowed NIOSH to significantly increase the CBRN respirator certification fee schedule because of the high costs of the live agent testing that is required.[3] However, only a small percentage of CBRN fees are remitted to NIOSH. Consequently, similar to the certification of other respirators, CBRN certification is not self-sustaining. The PPT Program is in the early phases of a plan to update the certification fee schedule for all types of respirators, and the committee urges approval of a revised fee structure that would fully recover the costs of certification activities. When certification cost recovery becomes a reality, it will be important that standards-setting efforts—and, most importantly, the expanded research program—are viewed as distinct activities, funded independently and in proportion to their contributions to worker safety and health.

The product and site audit programs are important tools to ensure manufacturer compliance as required by 42 CFR 84. The product audit program, in which respirators are routinely selected for testing from normal sales and distribution outlets, conducts only 40 to 60 product audit evaluations per year—a number that does not yield a statistically significant sample. The sampling strategy for this program needs to be carefully examined to ensure methodologically and statistically sound results. The site audit program is designed to ensure that manufacturers maintain quality facilities, processes, and products (see Chapter 2). A thoroughly monitored site audit program is needed to ensure that the audits, whether undertaken by PPT Program staff or by outside contractors, are conducted using valid methodology and appropriate data analysis.

Product recalls and product defect information are currently posted on the PPT Program's website. The committee acknowledges the importance of the detailed information that is posted but is concerned about the passive nature of the dissemination process. Without an effective means of disseminating this information, employers or employees might unknowingly be using products deemed ineffective. The current system for respirator certification does not include provisions for having devices "registered" (e.g., with purchasers' contact information), which

---

[2]The certification cost is a one-time cost for each type of respirator submitted for testing. After receiving certification, the manufacturer can produce hundreds to millions of that type of product, and therefore the certification costs are spread out over many items.

[3]CBRN respirator testing is conducted in part by the U.S. Department of Defense using live chemical warfare agents as part of the required testing.

undermines recall effectiveness. The PPT Program and manufacturers should have a direct and online method for contacting employers and others who purchase respirators in order to provide them with notices indicating that a problem or recall has occurred. It should be noted that the Mine Safety and Health Administration (MSHA) has recently begun requiring registration of self-contained self-rescuers (SCSRs) with mine operators. Other potential models include the registration card systems used for many consumer products. Review and adoption of best practices from the Consumer Product Safety Commission should be considered, as should instituting measures of recall effectiveness.

The NIOSH website currently provides the Certified Equipment List, a list of the respirators that have passed the certification process (NIOSH, 2008a). Providing certification test result data on the website would also be helpful to purchasers so that they can examine results on specific measures (e.g., breathing resistance).

INCREASE RESEARCH ON THE USE AND USABILITY OF PPT

Recommendation 4: Increase Research on the Use and Usability of PPT

The PPT Program should intensify its research directed at barriers to and facilitators of PPT use by workers. Such research should examine human factors and ergonomics, as well as individual behaviors and organizational behaviors, particularly workplace safety culture.

One of the greatest challenges to PPT effectiveness is ensuring that the worker is wearing the equipment and is wearing it correctly. Understanding that comfort is fundamentally a *safety* issue is a necessary prerequisite to improvement of the materials, design, and engineering of PPT in such a way that critically important human factors are taken into account. Improving usability will require research that focuses on task- and worker-centered design and a more in-depth knowledge of physiologic burdens (often heat stress) resulting from wearing PPT in the work environment. The PPT Program is moving forward in its work with the National Fire Protection Association and other partners in addressing these issues, particularly as they relate to physiologic burdens for emergency responders and firefighters. However, similar efforts are needed to assess usability issues for the majority of the workforce employed in other occupations. Collaborations with other NIOSH efforts in this area, particularly the work on Research to Practice and on Prevention through Design will be valuable as well as external collaborations.

Other important underinvestigated areas include behavior and the induction of behavioral change—specifically, changes by employers, work site managers, and workers that are essential prerequisites to increasing adherence to PPT protocols.

Research directions in this area should focus on improving the safety culture of organizations and individuals—a complex set of issues that involve training, leadership, and clarification of work site practices and policies (IOM, 2008).

ASSESS PPT USE AND EFFECTIVENESS IN THE WORKPLACE

Recommendation 5: Assess PPT Use and Effectiveness in the Workplace Using a Life-Cycle Approach

The PPT Program, in collaboration with relevant NIOSH divisions and other partners, should oversee an ongoing surveillance and field testing program to assess PPT use and effectiveness in the workplace. These efforts should emphasize a life-cycle approach by including both pre-market and interval post-market testing of PPT and include data collection on issues ranging from training to decontamination. Enhanced efforts would

- **Assess and critically appraise PPT use and effectiveness across all types of PPT (e.g., gloves, eye protection, respirators) and across relevant industry sectors and workplace environments;**
- **Require random periodic field testing of an adequately sized sample of PPT to assess effectiveness, usability, and durability with reasonable accuracy and precision; and**
- **Build on existing government and private-sector surveys and surveillance activities that collect PPT-relevant data and facilitate linkages to other datasets.**

Improvements in PPT will be driven both by efficacy data generated in the laboratory and effectiveness data gathered with equal scientific rigor in the workplace. Research priorities for PPT should be based on the prevalence and degree of exposure, modified by the strength of the observed association between these attributes of exposure and long- and short-term outcomes of illness and injury. The committee urges the NIOSH PPT Program to assess the effectiveness and use of PPT in the workplace across all phases of the lifetime of the products. This type of evaluation and surveillance construct could involve an array of approaches and methodologies, including pre- and post-market field testing of PPT products, surveys, on-site observations, focus groups and other end user inputs, as well as outcome and impact evaluations and formal cost-benefit analysis. Obtaining input from the end user of PPT products is particularly important.

In considering how best to plan and learn from a life cycle approach to data collection that will involve field testing and ongoing surveillance, it will be important to keep in mind that the immediate goals will differ with pre- and post-market field testing focused on the effectiveness of a specific product and surveillance focused on an ongoing assessment of PPT use. The committee believes these efforts are a necessary and vital investment for improving PPT and protecting workers from hazardous exposures. By choosing the appropriate methodologies and by building on current data collection efforts, sound investments can be made in obtaining data that are representative of workplace use and useful in improving PPT products and training.

With current limits on resources available for certification testing, virtually all of the product testing is now confined to the laboratory. Normal use is simulated in the laboratory, and consideration is given to testing under conditions that mimic workplace wear and tear on the product. However, the committee believes that more testing and research needs to be conducted in the field under workplace conditions with workers who depend on the sustained effectiveness of their PPT. The goal is an iterative improvement process that would include pre- and post-market testing plus utilization of other data sources including worker and employer feedback, surveillance, Health Hazard Evaluations (HHEs), and product and site audits. Further, field testing should occur during both the pre-marketing and post-marketing phases. For respirators and some other types of PPT, various pre-marketing certification tests could incorporate a field testing component. For other types of PPT that do not currently undergo a certification process by NIOSH, combined laboratory and field testing overseen by the PPT Program are necessary logical and scientific prerequisites to declaring PPT components and ensembles effective in the workplace.

Along the continuum of the life-cycle approach, decontamination, serviceability, and reusability issues need to be considered (IOM, 2006, 2008), especially for expensive and highly specialized CBRN equipment or for circumstances that could require extensive use of PPT, such as an influenza pandemic. Limited research efforts examining the safe decontamination and use of PPT are ongoing, but many important engineering and behavioral questions remain unanswered. Further research is also needed to define the trade-offs between disposing of and decontaminating PPT.

The PPT Program is currently developing a long-term surveillance action plan that was available to the committee in draft form in early March 2008 (NIOSH, 2008b; Chapter 3). Up to this point, most of the PPT Program's surveillance focus has been on inhalation exposure and respirator usage. For example, the PPT Program worked with the Bureau of Labor Statistics on the survey *Respirator Usage in Private Sector Firms* (BLS and NIOSH, 2003). Follow-up efforts to this survey included an assessment by a National Research Council (NRC) committee that resulted in the report *Measuring Respirator Use in the Workplace* (NRC, 2007). The

NRC report provided a number of recommendations for improvement of future PPT surveillance efforts.

Congruent with other recommendations addressing the future needs of the PPT Program, the committee urges that surveillance efforts extend beyond respirators and encompass all types of PPT. A sector-by-sector approach to surveying hazards and personal protective practices may be more efficient, cost-effective, and manageable than a large-scale survey of all workplaces. Although the proposed National PPT Program need not carry out all surveillance across all work sectors, consistent with the committee's prior recommendations on research, certification, and standards setting, it should have oversight responsibilities to ensure that the surveillance methods are coordinated and focused on relevant PPT issues. Developing a highly relevant PPT surveillance program, that incorporates long-term physiological endpoints, can best be coordinated across the NIOSH matrix of work sectors through the oversight of the expanded PPT Program.

Utilizing available data collection mechanisms could be useful in gathering information in the workplace and providing realistic assessments of how PPT is being used. For example, agreements with OSHA and MSHA might allow some gathering of data on the use of chemical protective clothing and other PPT based on inspections, through a sample survey of inspectors' findings. Collection of workplace data through a coordinated effort with the HHE Program might also prove fruitful. What is needed for true effectiveness research is information gathered from users and from direct observation and surveillance of PPT use in the workplace.

The PPT Program has been proactive in involving stakeholders in the development of changes to standards. Continued use of focus groups is critical to surveillance activity targeted at gaining insights into how PPT products are working and being used in the field. The committee emphasizes data collection on the effectiveness and use of PPT products as a priority for improving the protection afforded through PPT.

CONCLUDING REMARKS

The committee urges NIOSH to reexamine its commitment to PPT with a focus that is directly proportional to its importance to the safety and health of the millions of workers in the many workplaces where administrative and engineering controls are inadequate, impractical, or simply nonexistent.

NIOSH's Personal Protective Technology Program has made significant strides in improving the PPT available to workers, especially respiratory PPT. It is the committee's hope that the recommendations in this report will provide the necessary impetus for the development of a National Personal Protective Technology Program that conducts, coordinates, and provides national oversight of research, standards setting, and certification for all components of PPT and the interface between and among those components. The committee concludes, on the basis of all available evidence, that increasing the protection of workers from hazardous workplace exposures through the development and deployment of improved personal protective technologies is not only a critically important and worthwhile goal for workers in the United States and around the world but, with additional resources and thoughtful reorganization, is by no means out of reach.

REFERENCES

BLS (Bureau of Labor Statistics) and NIOSH (National Institute for Occupational Safety and Health). 2003. *Respirator usage in private sector firms, 2001.* http://www.cdc.gov/niosh/docs/respsurv/ (accessed January 22, 2008).

DHS (Department of Homeland Security). 2008. *Homeland Security Centers of Excellence.* http://www.dhs.gov/xres/programs/editorial_0498.shtm (accessed March 8, 2008).

IOM (Institute of Medicine). 2006. *Reusability of facemasks during an influenza pandemic.* Washington, DC: The National Academies Press.

IOM. 2008. *Preparing for an influenza pandemic: Personal protective equipment for healthcare workers.* Washington, DC: The National Academies Press.

NIOSH. 2008a. *Certified equipment list.* http://www.cdc.gov/niosh/npptl/topics/respirators/cel/ (accessed March 7, 2008).

NIOSH. 2008b. *PPT surveillance program action plan. Draft, March 5, 2008* (available through the National Academies Public Access File).

NRC (National Research Council). 2007. *Measuring respirator use in the workplace.* Washington, DC: The National Academies Press.

A

Framework for the Review of Research Programs of the National Institute for Occupational Safety and Health*

This is the second version of a document prepared by the National Academies Committee for the Review of NIOSH Research Programs[1] also referred to as the Framework Committee. This document is not a formal report of the National Academies—rather, it is a framework proposed for use by multiple National Academies evaluation committees to review up to 15 National Institute for Occupational Safety and Health (NIOSH) research programs. It is a working document subject to modification by the Framework Committee on the basis of responses received from evaluation-committee members, NIOSH, stakeholders, and the general public during the course of the assessments.

---

*Version of 8/10/07.

[1] Members of the committee at the time this version was produced were David Wegman, *Chair* (University of Massachusetts Lowell School of Health and Environment), William Bunn III (International Truck and Engine Corporation), Carlos Camargo (Harvard Medical School), Susan Cozzens (Georgia Institute of Technology), Letitia Davis (Massachusetts Department of Public Health), James Dearing (Kaiser Permanente-Colorado), Fred Mettler, Jr. (University of New Mexico School of Medicine), Franklin Mirer (Hunter College School of Health Sciences), Jacqueline Nowell (United Food and Commercial Workers International Union), Raja Ramani (Pennsylvania State University), Jorma Rantanen (International Commission on Occupational Health), Rosemary Sokas (University of Illinois at Chicago School of Public Health), Richard Tucker (Tucker and Tucker Consultants, Inc. and University of Texas at Austin), and James Zuiches (North Carolina State University). Sammantha Magsino (National Academies staff) was the study director. Joseph Wholey (University of Southern California), former committee member, contributed to the first version of this document. Part V includes brief biographies of current committee members.

This version reflects several significant changes to the original framework document (version 12/19/05) that was used to guide the work of the first four evaluation committees (Hearing Loss; Mining; Agriculture, Forestry, and Fishing; and Respiratory Disease). Changes were made in response to feedback from members and staff of these committees, as well as other comments on the original framework, in order to make the document more useful to evaluation committees as they carry out their work. In particular, the following changes were made to the framework document during the revision process:

- The wording of some of the relevance and impact scores were edited to make the wording more precise and to reduce situations where the original scores were non-unique or overlapping (revised scoring criteria are given in Boxes 2 and 3).
- A new table was added to provide explicit guidance to evaluation committees on how to weigh differences in the observed levels of "research priority" and "engagement in appropriate transfer activities" in arriving at a single integer score for relevance (see Table 6).
- The guidance on scoring was clarified to make more explicit that all scores are to be given as integers.
- The NIOSH logic model was updated (see Figure 1).
- The table on evaluation committee information needs (Table 2) was reorganized to be more consistent with the NIOSH logic model, and additional information needs identified by the first set of evaluation committees were added.
- A worksheet to assist with the development of scores has been deleted and key components of the worksheet have been incorporated into appropriate sections throughout the document.
- The organization of the document was modified to more closely follow the revised statement of task and to improve readability.
- A number of sections of text originally presented in outline form were modified in tables or boxes to make the information more accessible.

This second version of the framework document remains a working document subject to further modification by the Framework Committee on the basis of input received from evaluation committee members, NIOSH, stakeholders, and the general public during the course of the assessments.

APPENDIX A

CONTENTS

Abbreviations and Acronyms
 I. Introduction
   I.A. Overview of Charge to Evaluation Committees
   I.B. Evaluation Committees
   I.C. NIOSH Strategic Goals and Operational Plan
   I.D. Evaluation Committees' Information Needs
   I.E. Prior Evaluations
 II. Summary of Evaluation Process
   II.A. The Evaluation Flowchart (Figure 2)
   II.B. Steps in Program Evaluation
III. Evaluation of a NIOSH Research Program—The Process
   III.A. Analysis of External Factors Relevant to the NIOSH Research Program
   III.B. Evaluating NIOSH Research Programs by Using the Flowchart
     III.B.1. Identifying the Period for Evaluation
     III.B.2. Identifying Major Challenges (Figure 2, Circle)
     III.B.3. Analysis of Research-Program Strategic Goals and Objectives (Figure 2, Box A)
     III.B.4. Review of Inputs (Figure 2, Box B)
     III.B.5. Review of Activities (Figure 2, Box C)
     III.B.6. Review of Outputs (Figure 2, Box D)
     III.B.7. Review of Intermediate Outcomes (Figure 2, Box E)
     III.B.8. Review of End Outcomes (Figure 2, Box F)
     III.B.9. Review of Potential Outcomes
     III.B.10. Summary Evaluation Ratings and Rationale
   III.C. Assessment of NIOSH Process for Targeting Priority Research Needs and Committee Assessment of Emerging Issues
IV. Evaluation Committee Report Template

Figure 1   The NIOSH operational plan presented as a logic model
Figure 2   Flowchart for the evaluation of the NIOSH research program

Table 1   NORA High-Priority Research by Category
Table 2   Evaluation Committee Information Needs
Table 3   Examples of NIOSH Program Research and Transfer Activities
Table 4   Examples of Research-Program Outputs to Be Considered
Table 5   Background Context for Program Relevance and Impact
Table 6   Guidance for Weighting Research Priority and Engagement in Appropriate Transfer Activities in the Application of Relevance Score

Table 7	Targeting of New Research and Identification of Emerging Issues
Box 1	The Evaluation Process
Box 2	Scoring Criteria for Relevance
Box 3	Scoring Criteria for Impact
Box 4	Suggested Outline for Evaluation Committee Reports

Appendix A

ABBREVIATIONS AND ACRONYMS

ABLES	Adult Blood Lead Epidemiology and Surveillance
AOEC	Association of Occupational and Environmental Clinics
BLS	Bureau of Labor Statistics
CDC	Centers for Disease Control and Prevention
CSTE	Council of State and Territorial Epidemiologists
DOD	U.S. Department of Defense
EC	Evaluation Committee
EPA	Environmental Protection Agency
FACE	Fatality Assessment Control and Evaluation
FC	Framework Committee
HHE	Health Hazard Evaluation
MSHA	Mine Safety and Health Administration
NIH	National Institutes of Health
NIOSH	National Institute for Occupational Safety and Health
NORA	National Occupational Research Agenda
NORA1	National Occupational Research Agenda 1996-2005
NORA2	National Occupational Research Agenda 2005-forward
OSH Review Commission	Occupational Safety and Health Review Commission
OSHA	Occupational Safety and Health Administration
OSHAct	Occupational Safety and Health Act of 1970
PART	Performance Assessment Rating Tool
PEL	permissible exposure limit
RFA	request for applications
SENSOR	Sentinel Event Notification System of Occupational Risks

TMT	tools, methods, or technologies
USDA	U.S. Department of Agriculture

APPENDIX A

I. INTRODUCTION

In September 2004, the National Institute for Occupational Safety and Health (NIOSH) contracted with the National Academies to conduct a review of NIOSH research programs. The goal of this multiphase effort is to assist NIOSH in increasing the impact of its research efforts that are aimed at reducing workplace illnesses and injuries and improving occupational safety and health. The National Academies assigned the task to the Division on Earth and Life Studies and the Institute of Medicine.

The National Academies appointed a committee of 14 members, including persons with expertise in occupational medicine and health, industrial health and safety, industrial hygiene, epidemiology, civil and mining engineering, sociology, program evaluation, communication, and toxicology; representatives of industry and of the workforce; and a scientist experienced in international occupational-health issues. The Committee on the Review of NIOSH Research Programs, referred to as the Framework Committee (FC), prepared the first version of this document during meetings held on May 5-6, July 7-8, and August 15-16, 2005. This second version was finalized after the Framework Committee's May 30-31, 2007 meeting, based on feedback received on the framework from the first two independent evaluation committees, NIOSH leadership, and National Academies' staff, as well as discussions during an earlier FC meeting in April 2006.

This document is not a report of the National Academies; rather, it presents the evaluation framework developed by the FC to guide and provide common structure for the reviews of as many as 15 NIOSH programs during a 5-year period by independent evaluation committees (ECs) appointed by various divisions and boards of the National Academies. It is a working document to be shared with NIOSH and the public. This version has been modified by the FC on the basis of responses from the ECs, NIOSH, NIOSH stakeholders, and the public; and it may be modified again. It is incumbent on the ECs to consult with the FC if portions of the evaluation framework presented here are inappropriate for specific programs under review.

I.A. Overview of Charge to Evaluation Committees

At the first meeting of the FC, Lewis Wade, NIOSH senior science adviser, emphasized that a review of a NIOSH program should focus on the program's relevance to and impact on health and safety in the workplace. In developing a framework, the FC considered the following elements of the charge to the ECs:

1. Assessment of the program's contribution, through occupational safety and health research, to reductions in workplace hazardous exposures, illnesses, or injuries through

    a. an assessment of the relevance of the program's activities to the improvement of occupational safety and health, and
    b. an evaluation of the impact that the program's research has had in reducing work-related hazardous exposures, illnesses, and injuries.

    The evaluation committee will rate the performance of the program for its relevance and impact using an integer score of 1-5. Impact may be assessed directly (for example, on the basis of reductions in illnesses or injuries) or, as necessary, by using intermediate outcomes to estimate impact. Qualitative narrative evaluations should be included to explain the numerical ratings.
2. Assessment of the program's effectiveness in targeting new research areas and identifying emerging issues in occupational safety and health most relevant to future improvements in workplace protection. The committee will provide a qualitative narrative assessment of the program's efforts and suggestions about emerging issues that the program should be prepared to address.

I.B. Evaluation Committees

Individual ECs will be formed in accordance with the rules of the National Academies for the formation of balanced committees. Each EC will comprise persons with expertise appropriate for the specific NIOSH research program under review and may include representatives of stakeholder groups (such as labor unions and industry), experts in technology and knowledge transfer, and program evaluation. The EC will gather appropriate information from the sponsor (the NIOSH research program under review), stakeholders affected directly by NIOSH program research, and relevant independent parties. Each EC will consist of about 10 members, will meet about three times, and will prepare a report. The National Academies will deliver the report to NIOSH within 9 months of the first meeting of the EC. EC reports are subject to the National Academies report-review process.

I.C. NIOSH Strategic Goals and Operational Plan

As a prelude to understanding the NIOSH strategic goals and operational plan, NIOSH research efforts should be understood in the context of the Occupational

Safety and Health Act (OSHAct), under which it was created. The OSHAct identifies workplace safety and health as having high national priority and gives employers the responsibility for controlling hazards and preventing workplace injury and illness. The act creates an organizational framework for doing that, assigning complementary roles and responsibilities to employers and employees, the Occupational Safety and Health Administration (OSHA), the states, the Occupational Safety and Health (OSH) Review Commission, and NIOSH. The act recognizes NIOSH's role and responsibilities to be supportive and indirect. NIOSH research, training programs, criteria, and recommendations are intended to be used to inform and assist those more directly responsible for hazard control (OSHAct Sections 2b, 20, and 22).

Section 2b of the OSHAct describes 13 interdependent means of accomplishing the national goal, one of which is "by providing for research . . . and by developing innovative methods . . . for dealing with occupational safety and health problems." Sections 20 and 22 give the responsibility for that research to NIOSH. NIOSH is also given related responsibilities, including the development of criteria to guide prevention of work-related injury or illness; development of regulations for reporting on employee exposures to harmful agents; establishment of medical examinations, programs, or tests to determine illness incidence and susceptibility; publication of a list of all known toxic substances; assessment of potential toxic effects or risks associated with workplace exposure in specific settings; and conduct of education programs for relevant professionals to carry out the OSHAct purposes. NIOSH is also responsible for assisting the secretary of labor regarding education programs for employees and employers in hazard recognition and control.

The NIOSH mission is "to provide national and world leadership to prevent work-related illness, injury, disability, and death by gathering information, conducting scientific research, and translating the knowledge gained into products and services." To fulfill its mission, NIOSH has established the following strategic goals:[2]

- **Goal 1: Conduct research to reduce work-related illnesses and injuries.**
    - Track work-related hazards, exposures, illnesses, and injuries for prevention.
    - Generate new knowledge through intramural and extramural research programs.

---

[2] See http://www.cdc.gov/niosh/docs/strategic/.

- Develop innovative solutions for difficult-to-solve problems in high-risk industrial sectors.

- **Goal 2: Promote safe and healthy workplaces through interventions, recommendations, and capacity building.**
  - Enhance the relevance and utility of recommendations and guidance.
  - Transfer research findings, technologies, and information into practice.
  - Build capacity to address traditional and emerging hazards.

- **Goal 3: Enhance global workplace safety and health through international collaborations.**
  - Take a leadership role in developing a global network of occupational health centers.
  - Investigate alternative approaches to workplace illness and injury reduction and provide technical assistance to put solutions in place.
  - Build global professional capacity to address workplace hazards through training, information sharing, and research experience.

In 1994, NIOSH embarked on a national partnership effort to identify research priorities to guide occupational health and safety research for the next decade. The National Occupational Research Agenda (NORA) identified 21 high-priority research subjects (see Table 1). The NORA was intended not only for NIOSH but for the entire occupational health community. In the second decade of the NORA, NIOSH is working with its partners to update the research agenda, using an approach based on industry sectors. NIOSH and its partners are working through sector research councils to establish sector-specific research goals and objectives. The emphasis is on moving research to practice in workplaces through sector-based partnerships.

Figure 1 is the NIOSH operational plan, presented as a logic model,[3] of the path from inputs to outcomes for each NIOSH research program. The FC adapted the model to develop its framework. NIOSH will provide similar logic models appropriate to each research program evaluated by an EC.

---

[3]Developed by NIOSH with the assistance of the RAND Corporation.

TABLE 1 NORA High-Priority Research by Category

Category	Priority Research Area
Disease and injury	Allergic and irritant dermatitis
	Asthma and chronic obstructive pulmonary disease
	Fertility and pregnancy abnormalities
	Hearing loss
	Infectious diseases
	Low-back disorders
	Musculoskeletal disorders of upper extremities
	Trauma
Work environment and workforce	Emerging technologies
	Indoor environment
	Mixed exposures
	Organization of work
	Special populations at risk
Research tools and approaches	Cancer research methods
	Control technology and personal protective equipment
	Exposure-assessment methods
	Health-services research
	Intervention-effectiveness research
	Risk-assessment methods
	Social and economic consequences of workplace illness and injury
	Surveillance research methods

I.D. Evaluation Committees' Information Needs

Each NIOSH program under review will provide information to the relevant EC, including that outlined in Table 2. The EC may request additional information of NIOSH as needed, and NIOSH should provide it as quickly as is practical. NIOSH should consider organizing the information listed in Table 2 by subprogram or program as appropriate and to the extent possible.

In addition to the information provided by NIOSH, the EC should independently collect additional information that it deems necessary for evaluation (for example, the perspectives of stakeholders, such as OSHA, MSHA, unions and workforces, and industry). In conducting the review, the EC should continually examine how individual projects or activities contribute to the impact and relevance of a program as a whole.

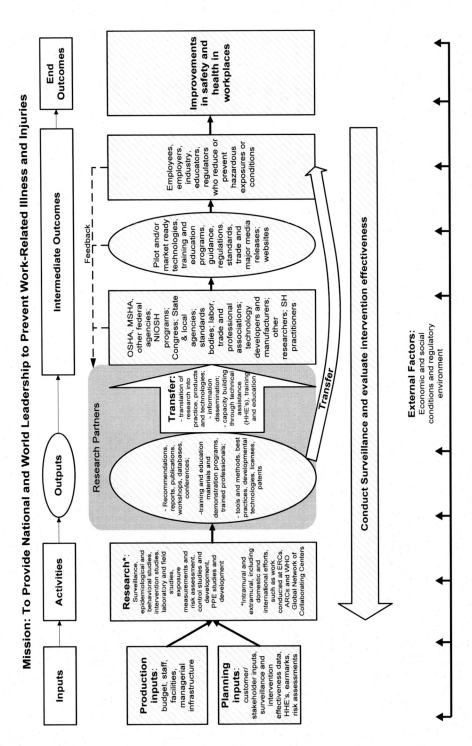

FIGURE 1 The NIOSH operational plan presented as a logic model.

APPENDIX A

TABLE 2 Evaluation Committee Information Needs

- **Program background and resources:**
  - Program history.
  - Major program challenges.
  - Program strategic goals and objectives, past (for period under review) and current.
  - Major subprograms (if appropriate).
  - Results of previous program reviews (for example, annual review by NIOSH leadership team or external scientific program reviews).
  - External factors affecting the program.

- **Interactions with stakeholders and with other NIOSH programs:**
  - The role of program research staff in NIOSH policy-setting, OSHA and MSHA standard-setting, voluntary standard-setting and other government policy functions.
  - Interactions and working relationships with other NIOSH programs.
  - Identification of other institutions and research programs with overlapping or similar portfolios and an explanation of the relationship between NIOSH activities and those of other institutions.
  - Key partnerships with employers, labor, other government organizations, academic institutions, nonprofit organizations, and international organizations.

- **Program inputs:**
  - Program resources (also called *production inputs*).
    - Funding by year for period under review.
    - Funding by objective or subprogram.
    - Program staffing, FTE's, and laboratory facilities, by subprogram (if indicated).
    - Percentage of program budget that is discretionary (beyond salaries).
    - Percentage of program budget that is earmarked.
    - Contributions from other agencies (in kind or funds).
  - Planning inputs.
    - Surveillance data, inputs from the Health Hazard Evaluation (HHE) or Fatality Assessment Control and Evaluation (FACE) program, or intramural and extramural research findings that influenced program goals and objectives.
    - Planning inputs from stakeholders, for example, advisory groups, NORA teams, and professional, industry, and labor groups (specify if any input from groups representing small business or vulnerable populations).
    - Related OSHA, Mine Safety and Health Administration (MSHA) strategic plans, or other input.
    - Process for soliciting and approving intramural research ideas.
    - Process for soliciting and approving program-supported extramural research activities.

- **Program activities (more details provided in Table 3):**
  - Intramural.
    - Surveillance activities.
    - Research activities (projects).

continued

TABLE 2 Continued

- Transfer activities to encourage implementation of research results for improved occupational safety and health (for example, information dissemination, technical assistance, and technology and knowledge transfer).
  - Key collaborations in intramural activities (for example, with other government agencies, academe, industry, and unions).
- Extramural funded by NIOSH.
  - Requests for applications (RFAs) developed by program.
  - Funded projects: grants, cooperative agreements, and contracts, such as
    ◊ Surveillance activities.
    ◊ Research activities.
    ◊ Transfer activities.
    ◊ Capacity-building activities.

- **Outputs (products of the research program—more details provided in Table 4):**
  - Intramural.
    - Peer-reviewed publications, agency reports, alerts, and recommendations.
    - Databases, Web sites, tools, and methods (including education and training materials).
    - Technologies developed and patents.
    - Sponsored conferences and workshops.
  - Extramural (to the extent practical).

- **Intermediate outcomes:**
  - Standards or guidelines issued by other agencies or organizations based in whole or in part on NIOSH research.
  - Adoption and use of control or personal protective technologies developed by NIOSH.
  - Evidence of industry, employer, or worker behavioral changes in response to research outputs.
  - Use of NIOSH products by workers, industry, occupational health and safety professionals, health care providers, and so on (including internationally).
  - NIOSH Web-site hits and document requests.
  - Unique staff or laboratory capabilities that serve as a national resource.
  - Other intermediate outcomes.

- **End outcomes:**
  - Data on program impact on rates and numbers of injuries and illnesses and exposures in the workplace (including trend data, if available).
  - Documentation of workplace risk reduction (quantitative, qualitative, or both).

- **Description of current processes for setting research priorities and identifying emerging issues in the workplace.**

I.E. Prior Evaluations

Several NIOSH programs have already been evaluated by internal and external bodies. The evaluations may have been part of an overall assessment of NIOSH, such as the 2005 Performance Assessment Rating Tool (PART) review,[4] or the evaluation of specific research program elements, such as any external scientific-program review. NIOSH should inform of, and the ECs should review, all prior evaluations of the program under review as an aid to understanding the evolution of the program and its elements. The EC evaluations, however, are independent of prior reviews and evaluations.

II. SUMMARY OF EVALUATION PROCESS

The ECs will assess the relevance and impact of NIOSH research programs. In conducting their evaluations, the ECs should ascertain whether NIOSH is doing the right things (relevance) and whether these things are improving health and safety in the workplace (impact).

II.A. The Evaluation Flowchart
(Figure 2)

To address its charge, the FC simplified the logic model of Figure 1 into a flowchart (Figure 2) that breaks the NIOSH logic model into discrete, sequential program components to be assessed by the EC. Each component of Figure 2 is addressed in greater detail in the indicated section of this document. The FC understands that the activities of any research program will not be as linear as presented in either Figures 1 or 2. The major components to be evaluated are

- major program *challenges,*
- strategic *goals and objectives,*
- *inputs* (such as budget, staff, facilities, the institute's research management, the NIOSH Board of Scientific Counselors, the NORA process, and NORA work groups),
- *activities* (efforts by NIOSH staff, contractors, and grantees, such as hazard surveillance; surveillance for injury, illness, and biomarkers of effect; exposure-measurement research; safety-systems research; injury-prevention research; health-effects research; intervention

---

[4]The PART focuses on assessing program-level performance and is one of the measures of success of the budget and performance integration initiative of the president's management agenda (see CDC Occupational Safety and Health at http://www.whitehouse.gov/omb/budget/fy2006/pma/hhs.pdf).

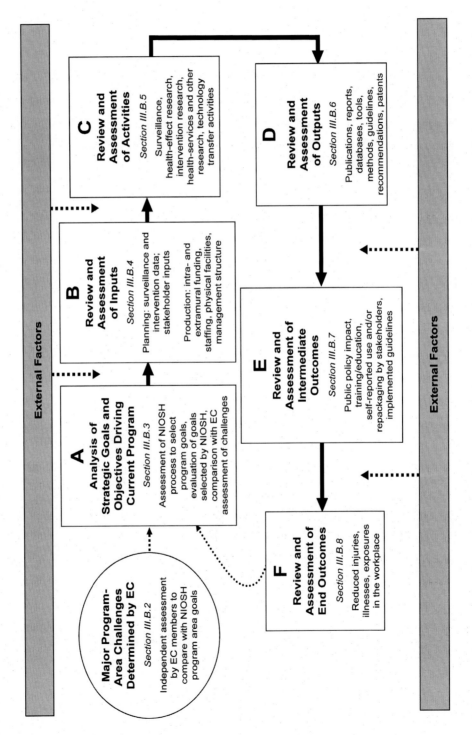

FIGURE 2 Flowchart for the evaluation of the NIOSH research program.

research; health-services research; and technology and knowledge transfer activities),
- *outputs* (NIOSH products, such as publications, reports, conferences, databases, tools, methods, guidelines, recommendations, education and training, and patents),
- *intermediate outcomes* (responses by NIOSH stakeholders to NIOSH products, such as public or private policy change, training and education in the form of workshop or seminar attendance, self-reported use or repackaging of NIOSH data by stakeholders, adoption of NIOSH-developed technologies, implemented guidelines, licenses, and reduction in workplace hazardous exposure), and
- *end outcomes* (such as reduction in work-related injuries or illnesses or hazardous exposures in the workplace).

The flowchart summarizes the FC's vision of how a program evaluation should occur. In evaluating each program or major subprogram, the EC must collect, analyze, and evaluate information on items described in each of the boxes of Figure 2, regardless of management structure (such as linear or matrix). The FC recognizes that the components of any program will not fit perfectly in any category in Figure 1 or 2. For example, training and development programs were appropriately defined as outputs by NIOSH in the logic model (Figure 1), but the FC finds more value in focusing on the responses to these outputs as intermediate outcomes (Figure 2, Box E) in the flowchart. The committee further recognizes that matrix organizations may have little control over the input portion of the logic model and that matrix program management may have fewer resources of its own on which to base its decisions. Following the suggested evaluation procedures, however, should ensure a desired level of consistency and comparability among all the ECs.

Drawing on the program logic model, the flowchart, and EC members' expertise, the ECs will delineate important inputs and external factors affecting the NIOSH research program's agenda and the consequences of NIOSH research activities. Examples of external factors are research activities of industry and other federal agencies and the political and regulatory environment. For purposes of this review, the results of inputs and external factors are the program research activities, outputs, and associated transfer activities that may result in intermediate outcomes and possibly end outcomes.

II.B. Steps in Program Evaluation

The FC concludes that useful evaluation requires a disciplined focus on a small number of questions or hypotheses typically related to program goals, performance criteria, and performance standards; a rigorous method of answering the questions or testing the hypotheses; and a credible procedure for developing qualitative and quantitative assessments. The evaluation process developed by the FC is summarized in Box 1 and described in detail in Section III of this document.

III. EVALUATION OF A NIOSH RESEARCH PROGRAM—THE PROCESS

III.A. Analysis of External Factors Relevant to the NIOSH Research Program

As depicted in the logic model (Figure 1), reduction in injury and illness (end outcomes) or in exposure (intermediate outcome) is affected by stakeholder activities (external factors). Actions of those in labor, industry, regulatory entities, and others beyond NIOSH's control are necessary for the implementation of NIOSH recommendations. Implementation of research findings may depend on existing or future policy considerations.

External factors may be considered as forces beyond the control of NIOSH that may affect the evolution of a program. External factors influence NIOSH's progress through all phases of the logic model and flowchart; from inputs to end outcomes (see Figures 1 and 2). Identification of external factors by an EC is essential because it provides the context for evaluation of the NIOSH program. External factors may be best assessed on the basis of the expert judgment of EC members who have knowledge of the field of research. Information regarding external factors should also be sought from NIOSH, OSHA, and MSHA staff and from other stakeholders. The EC, however, may choose additional approaches to assess external factors. NIOSH should identify and describe external factors early in the evaluation sequence (see Table 2). Factors external to NIOSH might have been responsible for achieving some outcomes or might have presented formidable obstacles. The EC must address both possibilities.

Some external factors may involve constraints on research activities related to target populations, methodologic issues, and resource availability. ECs might examine whether or not the following are true:

- Projects addressing a critical health need are technologically feasible. However, a workforce of appropriate size and with appropriate duration and distribution of exposure for measuring a health effect may not exist; for example, no population of workers has been exposed for 30 years to formaldehyde at the current OSHA permissible exposure limit (PEL), so the related cancer mortality cannot yet be directly assessed.
- Research is inhibited because NIOSH investigators are unable to access an adequate study population. Under current policy, NIOSH must

> **BOX 1**
> **The Evaluation Process**
>
> 1. Gather appropriate information from NIOSH and other sources (see Table 2).
>
> 2. Determine timeframe to be covered in the evaluation (see III.B.1).
>
> 3. Identify major program area challenges and objectives (see III.B.2).
>   All NIOSH research programs are designed to be responsive to present or future workplace safety and health issues. Each research program should have its own objectives. Each EC will provide an independent assessment of the major workplace health and safety problems related to the program under review and determine whether they are consistent with the program's stated goals and objectives.
>
> 4. Identify subprograms and major projects in the research program.
>   Each EC must determine how to disaggregate a program to achieve a manageable and meaningful evaluation of its components, and of the overall program. A program may need to be broken down into several recognizable subprograms or major projects if an effective evaluation is to be organized. It may be advantageous for an EC to disaggregate a program into subprograms that NIOSH identifies.
>
> 5. Evaluate the subprogram components sequentially (see III.B.2 through III.B.8), using the flowchart (Figure 2) as a guide.
>   This will involve a qualitative assessment of each component of the research program. ECs will use professional judgment to answer questions and follow the guidance provided by the FC.
>
> 6. Evaluate the research program's potential outcomes that are not yet appreciated (see III.B.9).
>
> 7. Evaluate the important subprogram outcomes specifically for contributions to improvements in workplace safety and health.
>   Guidance is provided with specific items for consideration (see III.B.10).
>
> 8. Evaluate and score the overall program for *relevance* (see III.B.10).
>   Final program ratings will consist of an integer score and discussion of its rationale.
>
> 9. Evaluate and score the overall program for *impact* (see III.B.10).
>   Final program ratings will consist of an integer score and discussion of its rationale.
>
> 10. Identify success in targeting priority research and emerging issues (see III.C).
>   The EC should briefly discuss its assessment of the NIOSH program's process for determining priorities for research and emerging workplace issues. The ECs should also independently identify emerging workplace issues for which the NIOSH program under review should be prepared.
>
> 11. Prepare report by using the template provided in Section IV as a guide.

either obtain an invitation by management to study a workplace or seek a judicial order to provide authority to enter a worksite. (Cooperation under court order may well be insufficient for effective research.)
- Research is inhibited because the work environment, materials, and historical records cannot be accessed even with management and workforce cooperation.
- Adequate or established methods do not exist for assessing the environment.
- The NIOSH contribution to a particular field of research is reduced because other institutions are working in the same field.
- NIOSH resources are inadequate to tackle key questions.

Evaluation of the impact of NIOSH research outputs on worker health and safety may require consideration of external factors that might impede or aide implementation, measurement, and so on. ECs might consider whether or not the following are true:

- Regulatory end points are unachievable because of obstacles to regulation or because of differing priorities of the regulatory agencies. For example, there may be no implementation of recommendations for improved respiratory protection programs for health-care workers because of enforcement policies or lack of acceptance by the health-care institution administrators.
- A feasible control for a known risk factor or exposure is unimplemented because the costs of implementation are too high or because current economic incentives do not favor such actions.
- End outcomes are unobservable because baseline and continuing surveillance data are not available. For example, the current incidence of occupational noise-induced hearing loss is not known although surveillance for a substantial threshold shift is feasible. (NIOSH conducts surveillance of work-related illnesses, injuries, and hazards, but comprehensive surveillance is not possible with existing resources.)
- Reductions in adverse effects of chronic exposure cannot be measured. For example, 90% of identified work-related mortality is from diseases, such as cancer, that arise only after decades of latency after first exposure; therefore, effects of reducing exposure to a carcinogen cannot be observed in the timeframe of most interventions.
- A promulgated regulation requires a technology that was developed but not widely used.

- Reductions in fatal traumatic injuries occur because more-hazardous manufacturing jobs are replaced by less-hazardous knowledge-based jobs.

III.B. Evaluating NIOSH Research Programs by Using the Flowchart

The FC used the NIOSH logic model (Figure 1) to define the scope and stages of an EC evaluation. The evaluation of the elements in the flowchart (Figure 2) summarizes the FC's vision of how a program evaluation should proceed. FC members also identified numerous possible factors to consider in assessing the relevance of NIOSH research-program components, including the following:

- The severity or frequency of health and safety hazards addressed and the number of people at risk (magnitude) for these hazards.
- The extent to which NIOSH research programs identify and address gender-related issues and issues of vulnerable populations: Vulnerable populations are defined as groups of workers who have biologic, social, or economic characteristics that place them at increased risk for work-related conditions or on whom inadequate data have been collected. Vulnerable populations include disadvantaged minorities, disabled persons, low-wage workers, and non-English-speakers for whom language or other barriers present health or safety risks.
- The extent to which NIOSH research programs address the health and safety needs of small businesses.
- The "life stage" of problems being addressed: As the health effects are understood, efforts should shift to intervention research, from efficacy to intervention, and to intervention-effectiveness research. Gaps in the spectrum of prevention need to be addressed; for example, research on exposure assessment may be necessary before the next intervention steps can be taken.
- The structure, in addition to the content, of the research program: A relevant research program is more than a set of unrelated research projects; it is an integrated program involving interrelated surveillance, research, and transfer activities.
- Appropriate NIOSH consideration of stakeholder input.

The ECs may consider those and other important factors that bear on relevance as they progress through each stage of an evaluation.

The following subsections are intended to guide the EC through the evaluation process and flowchart in Figure 2. Each begins with a definition of the component being evaluated, provides questions for the EC to consider during the course of its evaluation, and provides some guidance regarding the assessment of the component. The FC admittedly provides little guidance regarding the evaluation of programs that are organized in a matrix structure or programs that have large extramural research components. Because of the uniqueness of each program, each EC must determine the most reasonable way to apply the criteria established in this document.

III.B.1 Identifying the Period for Evaluation

By studying materials presented by the NIOSH research program and other sources, the EC will become familiar with the history of the research program being evaluated and its major subprograms, goals, objectives, resources, and other pertinent information. Having that information, the EC should choose the period most appropriate for the evaluation. EC efforts should focus on the impact and relevance of the NIOSH program in the most recent appropriate period. As a starting point, the ECs might consider three general timeframes:

- 1970-1995, the period from the founding of NIOSH to the initiation of NORA (pre-NORA period)
- 1996-2005 (NORA 1 period)
- After 2005 (NORA 2 period)

Those timeframes are provided as general guidance; the period chosen for review will take into consideration suggestions from the NIOSH research program under review. It is recognized that many of the intermediate and end outcomes documented since 1996 are consequences of research outputs completed before 1996.

III.B.2 Identifying Major Challenges
(Figure 2, Circle)

Early in the assessment process, the EC itself should identify the major workplace health and safety challenges for the research program under review. In arriving at a list of challenges, the EC should rely on surveillance findings, including those of NIOSH investigations of sentinel events (through health-hazard or fatality-assessment programs), external advisory inputs, and its own expert judgment. The EC will then be able to compare its own assessment of workplace challenges with the NIOSH program goals and objectives. The congruence between the two will be useful during the assessment of relevance.

III.B.3. Analysis of Research-Program Strategic Goals and Objectives (Figure 2, Box A)

The research program goals and objectives should be evaluated with a focus on how each program goal is related to NIOSH's agency wide strategic goals and to the program challenges identified in the step above (Section III.B.2). The importance or relevance of an issue may differ from the influence of NIOSH-funded research in addressing it. The EC should recognize that NIOSH research priorities may be circumstantial (for example, congressionally funded) rather than based on NIOSH's assessment of the state of knowledge.

Questions to Guide the Evaluation Committee

1. Are the strategic goals and objectives of the program well defined and clearly described?
2. How well were program goals and objectives aligned with NORA 1 priorities during the last decade?
3. How are current program strategic goals and objectives related to current NIOSH strategy, including NORA 2?
4. Are the research program goals, objectives, and strategies relevant to the major challenges for the research program and likely to address emerging problems in the research program (as determined by the EC while addressing Section III.B.2)?
    a. Did past program goals and objectives (research and dissemination and transfer activities) focus on the most relevant problems and anticipate the emerging problems in the research program?
    b. Do the current program goals and objectives target the most relevant problems?

Assessment

The EC should provide a qualitative assessment that discusses the relevance of the program's goals, objectives, and strategies in relation to its major challenges.

III.B.4. Review of Inputs (Figure 2, Box B)

Planning inputs include input from stakeholders, surveillance and intervention data, and risk assessments. Production inputs include intramural and extramural funding, staffing, management structure, and physical facilities.

The EC should examine existing intramural and extramural resources and, potentially, prior surveys or case studies that might have been developed specifically to assess progress in reducing workplace illnesses and injuries and to provide information relevant to the targeting of research to future needs. The NIOSH research program should provide the EC all relevant planning and production inputs (see below and Table 2 for examples).

Planning Inputs

Planning inputs can be qualitative or quantitative. Sources of qualitative inputs include the following:

- Federal advisory committees (such as the Board of Scientific Counselors, the Mine Safety and Health Research Advisory Committee, and the National Advisory Committee on Occupational Safety and Health)
- NORA research partners, initial NORA stakeholder meetings, later NORA team efforts (especially strategic research plans), and the NORA Liaison Committee and federal liaison committee recommendations
- Industry, labor, academe, professional associations, industry associations, and the Council of State and Territorial Epidemiologists (CSTE)
- OSHA and MSHA strategic plans and other federal research agendas

Attention should be given to how comprehensive the inputs have been and to what extent gaps in input have been identified and considered by NIOSH.
Sources of quantitative inputs include the following:

- Intramural surveillance information, such as descriptive data on exposures and outcomes (appropriate data may be available from a number of NIOSH divisions and laboratories)
- HHEs
- Reports from the FACE program
- Extramural health-outcome and exposure-assessment data from OSHA, MSHA (both safety and health inspection data), the Bureau of Labor Statistics, the U.S. Department of Defense (DOD), and the US Department of Agriculture (USDA) (fatality, injury, and illness surveillance data); state government partners, including NIOSH-funded state surveillance programs, such as Sentinel Event Notification System of Occupational Risks (SENSOR), Adult Blood Lead Epidemiology and

Surveillance (ABLES), and state-based FACE; and nongovernment organizations, such as the National Safety Council, the Association of Occupational and Environmental Clinics (AOEC), the American Society of Safety Engineers, and the American College of Occupational and Environmental Medicine
- Appropriate data from investigator-initiated extramural research funded by NIOSH

Production Inputs

For the research program under review, NIOSH should identify portions of the NIOSH intramural budget, staff, facilities, and management that play major roles in the research program. Production inputs should be described primarily in terms of intramural research projects, relevant extramural projects (particularly cooperative agreements and contracts), HHEs, and related staff. Consideration should also be given to leveraged funds provided by such partners as the National Institutes of Health (NIH) and the Environmental Protection Agency (EPA) for joint requests for applications or program announcements; and to OSHA, MSHA, and U.S. Department of Defense (DOD) contracts with NIOSH.

Assessment of inputs should include EC consideration of the degree to which allocation of funding and personnel was commensurate with the resources needed to conduct the research and the extent to which funding for the relevant intramural research activity has been limited by lack of discretionary spending beyond salaries (travel, supplies, external laboratory services, and so on). Thus, assessments should consider the adequacy of the qualitative and quantitative planning and production inputs, given the tasks at hand.

Questions to Guide the Evaluation Committee

1. Do planning, production, and other input data promote program goals?
2. How well are major planning, production, and other program inputs used to support the major activities?
3. Is input obtained from stakeholders, including input representing vulnerable working populations and small businesses?
4. Are production inputs (intramural and extramural funding, staffing, management, and physical infrastructure resources) consistent with program goals and objectives?

Assessment

The EC should provide a qualitative assessment that discusses the quality, adequacy, and use of inputs.

III.B.5. Review of Activities
(Figure 2, Box C)

Activities are defined as the efforts and work of a program's staff, grantees, and contractors. For present purposes, activities of the NIOSH program under review are divided into research and transfer activities. Table 3 is intended to guide the EC and NIOSH as to the type and organization of information required to evaluate program activities. The table may be incomplete, and some types of research activity may not be applicable to a given NIOSH program. Research activities include safety research, health-outcomes research, safety-design research, and safety-systems research. Transfer activities include information dissemination, training, technical assistance, and education designed to translate research outputs into content and formats that are designed for application in the workplace. Depending on the scope of the program under review, activities may also be grouped by research-program objectives or subprograms.

Conventional occupational safety and health research focuses appropriately on injury, illness, or death; on biomarkers of exposure; and on health effects of new technology, personal protective equipment, and regulations. A focus on surveillance research may be needed when available data inputs are inadequate. A focus on socioeconomic and policy research and on diffusion research is also needed to effect change, because not all relevant intermediate outcomes occur in the workplace. NIOSH may be able to affect important outcomes farther out on the causal chain so as to influence health and safety in the workplace. Other research that might prove important in addressing NIOSH's mission includes the following:

- Surveillance research to assess the degree of significant or systematic underreporting of relevant injuries, illnesses, and biomarkers
- Socioeconomic research on cost-shifting between worker compensation and private insurance
- Research on methods to build health and safety capacity in community health centers that serve low-income or minority-group workers and to improve recognition and treatment of work-related conditions
- Transfer research to change health and safety knowledge of adolescents while they are in high school to improve the likelihood of reduced injuries as they enter the workforce

TABLE 3 Examples of NIOSH Program Research and Transfer Activities

Surveillance (including hazard and injury, illness, and biomarkers of exposure or effect health surveillance and evaluation of surveillance systems)

Health-effects research (illnesses, injuries, and biomarkers):
    Epidemiology
    Toxicology
    Physical and safety risk factors (laboratory-based)
    Development of clinical-screening methods and tools

Exposure-assessment research:
    Chemical hazards
    Physical hazards
    Biologic hazards
    Ergonomic hazards
    Safety (traumatic injury) hazards

Safer-design and safety-systems research

Intervention research:
    Control technologies
        Engineering controls and alternatives
        Administrative controls
        Personal protective equipment
    Work organization
    Community participation
    Policy (such as alternative approaches to targeting inspections)
    Design for safety
    Emergency preparedness and disaster response

Diffusion and dissemination research:
    Training effectiveness
    Information-dissemination effectiveness
    Diffusion of technology

Health-services and other research:
    Access to occupational health care
    Infrastructure—delivery of occupational-health services, including international health and safety
    Socioeconomic consequences of work-related injuries and illnesses
    Worker compensation

Technology-transfer and other transfer activities:
    Information dissemination
    Training programs
    Technical assistance

- Community-based participatory research on differences between recently arrived immigrants and U.S.-born workers regarding perceptions of acceptable health and safety risks so that programs can be targeted to meet the workforce training needs of immigrant workers

Transfer activities should be reviewed to determine whether the NIOSH program appropriately targets its outputs in a manner that will have the greatest impact. Ideally, information dissemination should be proactive, and strategic dissemination should be informed by research on the diffusion of new technologies, processes, and practices. Highly relevant information and technology transfer should include plans for appropriate transfer to all appropriate worker populations, including those considered vulnerable. Training should be incorporated into the strategic goals of all research fields where appropriate.

The EC should review project-level research and transfer activities (including surveillance activities) that have been completed, are in progress, or planned by the program under review. The program under review should provide a list of activities and specify whether they are intramural or extramural. For each extramural project, the key organizations and principal investigators' names should be requested, as should whether the project was in response to a request for proposal or a request for application. For each intramural project, the EC should ask NIOSH to provide a list of key collaborators (from another government agency, academe, industry, or unions).

The EC should evaluate each of the research activities outlined in Table 3 if it forms an important element of the program research. In the case of a sector-based research program (for example, mining or construction) in which health-effects research is not being reviewed, the EC should determine what research inputs influence the program's strategic goals and objective, and then assess the value of the inputs.

Questions to Guide the Evaluation Committee in Assessing Research Activities

1. What are the major subprograms or groupings of activities within the program?
2. Are activities consistent with program goals and objectives?
3. Are research activities relevant to the major challenges of the research program?
    a. Do they address the most serious outcomes?
    b. Do they address the most common outcomes?
    c. Do they address the needs of both sexes, vulnerable working populations, and small businesses?

4. Are research activities appropriately responsive to the input of stakeholders?
5. To what extent are partners involved in the research activities?
6. Are partners involved early in the research process so that they could participate in determining research objectives and research design?
7. Were original resource allocations appropriate for the research activities, and do they remain appropriate?
8. To what extent does peer reviews (internal, external, and midcourse) affect the activities?
9. Is there adequate monitoring of quality-assurance procedures to ensure credible research data, analyses, and conclusions?

Questions to Guide the Evaluation Committee in Assessing Transfer Activities
1. Is there a coherent planned program of transfer activities?
2. Are the program's information dissemination, training, education, technical assistance, or publications successful in reaching the workplace or relevant stakeholders in other settings? How widespread is the response?
3. To what degree have stakeholders responded to NIOSH information and training products?
4. Is there evidence that the formats for information products were selected in response to stakeholder preferences?
5. To what extent do program personnel rely on assessment of stakeholder needs and reactions to prototype information and training projects (formative evaluation techniques)?
6. To what extent does the program build research and education capacity internally and among stakeholders?

Assessment

For this part of the assessment, the EC will provide a qualitative assessment that discusses relevance. This assessment should include consideration of the external factors identified in Section III.A that constrain choices of research projects and the relevance and effectiveness of transfer activities. The EC should consider the appropriateness of resource allocations. A highly relevant program would address high-priority needs, produce high-quality results, be appropriately collaborative, be of value to stakeholders, and be substantially engaged in transfer activities. A program may be less relevant to the extent that those key elements are not up to the mark or are missing. The discussion should cover those aspects in sufficient detail to arrive at a qualitative assessment of the activities. Assessment of the transfer activities must include considerations of program planning, coherence, and impact. The EC might also consider the incorporation of international research results into NIOSH knowledge-transfer activities for industry sectors in the United States.

III.B.6. Review of Outputs
(Figure 2, Box D)

An output is a direct product of a NIOSH research program. Outputs may be designed for researchers, practitioners, intermediaries, and end-users, such as consumers. Outputs can be in the form of publications in peer-reviewed journals, recommendations, reports, Web-site content, workshops and presentations, databases, educational materials, scales and methods, new technologies, patents, technical assistance, and so on. Outputs of the research program's extramurally funded activities should also be considered. Table 4 lists examples of major outputs to be considered by the EC. The NIOSH research program should make every effort to include all pertinent data of the types listed in the table.

Outputs may be tailored to the intended audience to communicate information most effectively and increase the likelihood of comprehension, knowledge, attitude formation, and behavioral intent. The extent of use of formative evaluation data (data gathered before communication for the purpose of improving the likelihood of the intended effects) and the extent of intended user feedback in the design of the output can be considered indicators of appropriate quality assessment.

Some activities such as collaborations can also legitimately be conceptualized as outputs, because the collaboration itself is a result of NIOSH efforts. Cooperation, coordination, more intensive collaboration, and eventual formal partnering can be considered important outputs leading to desirable intermediate outcomes. Technology and knowledge transfer is greatly facilitated through such relationships. The extent of collaboration with other organizations in the determination of research agendas, the conduct of research, the dissemination of research results, and interorganization involvement in the production of outputs can all be measures of output quality and quantity. The EC may consider coauthorship while trying to determine the importance of NIOSH research to the broader research community.

The NIOSH program should provide information on all relevant outputs of the program under review produced during the chosen period.

Questions to Guide the Evaluation Committee

1. What are the major outputs of the research program?
2. Are output levels consistent with resources allocated (were resources allocated and used efficiently to produce outputs)?

TABLE 4 Examples of Research-Program Outputs to Be Considered

Peer-reviewed publications by NIOSH staff:
    Number of original research articles by NIOSH staff
    Number of review articles by NIOSH staff (including best-practices articles)
    Complete citation for each publication
    Complete copies of the "top five" articles
    Collaboration with other public- or private-sector researchers
    Publications in the field of interest with other support by investigators also funded by NIOSH (for example, ergonomic studies with other support by an investigator funded by NIOSH to do ergonomics work, in which case NIOSH should get some credit for seeding interest or drawing people into the field)

Peer-reviewed publications by external researchers funded by NIOSH:
    Number of NIOSH-funded original research articles by external researchers
    Number of NIOSH-funded review articles by external researchers (including best-practices articles)
    Complete citation for each written report
    Complete copies of the "top five" articles
    Collaboration with other government or academic researchers

NIOSH reports in the research program:
    Number of written reports
    Complete citation for each written report
    Complete copies of the "top five" reports

Sponsored conferences and workshops:
    Number of sponsored conferences
    Number of sponsored workshops
    Description of conferences and workshops (title, date, sponsors, target audience, number of participants, and resulting products)
    NIOSH's assessment of value or impact

Databases:
    Number of major databases created by NIOSH staff
    Number of major databases created by external researchers funded by NIOSH grants
    Description of databases:
        Title, objective (in one to four sentences), and start and stop dates
        Partial vs. complete sponsorship (if partial, who were cosponsors?)
        Study or surveillance-system design, study population, and sample size
        Primary "products" of the database (such as number of peer-reviewed articles and reports)
    Complete copies of the "top two" publications or findings, to date, from each database

continued

TABLE 4 Continued

Recommendations:
    Number of major recommendations
    Description of recommendations:
        Complete citation (article, report, or conference where recommendation was made)
        Summary in one to four sentences
        Percentage of target audience that has adopted recommendation 1, 5, and 10 years later
        Up to three examples of implementation in the field
    Identification of "top five" recommendations to date

Tools, methods, and technologies (TMT):
    Number of major TMT (includes training and education materials)
    Descriptions of TMT
        Title and objective of TMT (in one to four sentences)
        Complete citation (if applicable)
        Percentage of target audience that has used TMT 1, 5, and 10 years later
        Up to three examples of implementation in the field
    Identification of "top 5" TMT to date

Patents:
    Total number of patents
    For each:
        Title and objective (in one to four sentences)
        Complete citation
        Percentage of target audience that has used product 1, 5, and 10 years later
        Up to three examples of implementation in the field
    Identification of "top five" patents to date

Miscellaneous:
    Any other important program outputs

3. Does the research program produce outputs that address high-priority areas?
4. To what extent does the program generate important new knowledge or technology?
5. Are there widely cited peer-reviewed publications considered to report "breakthrough" results?
6. What, if any, internal or external capacity-building outputs are documented?
7. Are outputs relevant to both sexes, vulnerable populations, and do they address health disparities?
8. Are outputs relevant to health and safety problems of small businesses?

APPENDIX A

9. Are products user-friendly with respect to readability, simplicity, and design?
10. To what extent does the program help to build the internal or extramural institutional knowledge base?
11. Does the research produce effective cross-agency, cross-institute, or internal-external collaborations?
12. To what extent does the program build research and education capacity (internal or external)?

Assessment

The EC should provide a qualitative assessment discussing relevance and utility. The outputs of a highly ranked program will address needs in high-priority areas, contain new knowledge or technology that is effectively communicated, contribute to capacity-building inside and outside NIOSH, and be relevant to the pertinent populations. The discussion should cover those aspects in sufficient detail to support the qualitative assessment of the outputs.

III.B.7. Review of Intermediate Outcomes (Figure 2, Box E)

Intermediate outcomes are important indicators of stakeholder response to NIOSH outputs. They reflect the impact of program activities and may lead to the desired end outcome of improved workplace safety and health. Intermediate outcomes include the production by those outside of NIOSH of guidelines or regulations based wholly or partly on NIOSH research (products adopted as national or international public policy or as policy or guidelines by private organizations or industry); contributions to training and education programs sponsored by other organizations; use of publications or other materials by workers, industry, and occupational safety and health professionals in the field; and citations of NIOSH research by industrial and academic scientists.

Intermediate outcomes allow inference that a program's outputs are associated with observed changes in the workplace. Thus, an intermediate outcome reflects an assessment of worth by NIOSH stakeholders (such as managers in industrial firms) about NIOSH research or its products (for example, NIOSH training workshops). Intermediate outcomes that are difficult to monitor but may be valid indicators of relevance or utility include self-report measures by users of NIOSH outputs. Such indicators include the extent to which key intermediaries find value in NIOSH products or databases for the repackaging of health and safety information, the extent to which NIOSH recommendations are in place and attended to in workplaces, and employee or employer knowledge of and adherence to NIOSH-recommended practices.

Questions to Guide the Evaluation Committee

1. Do program outputs result in or contribute to stakeholder training or education activities used in the workplace or in school or apprentice programs? If so, how?
2. Do program activities and outputs result in regulations, public policy, or voluntary standards or guidelines that are transferred to or created by the workplace?
3. Has the program resulted in changes in employer or worker practices associated with the reduction of risk (for example, in the adoption of new feasible control or personal protective technologies or administrative control concepts)?
4. Does the program contribute to changes in health-care practices to improve recognition and management of occupational health conditions?
5. Does the program result in research partnerships with stakeholders that lead to changes in the workplace?
6. To what extent do the program's stakeholders find value in NIOSH products (as shown by document requests, Web-site hits, conference attendance, and so on)?
7. Does the program or a subprogram provide unique staff or laboratory capability that is a necessary national resource? If so, is it adequate, or does it need to be enhanced or reduced?
8. Has the program resulted in interventions that protect both sexes, vulnerable workers, or address the needs of small businesses?
9. To what extent did the program contribute to increased capacity at worksites to identify or respond to safety and health threats?

Assessment

Only a qualitative assessment of product development, usefulness, and impact is required at this point in the EC report. Some thought should be given to the relative value of intermediate outcomes, and the FC recommends applying the well-accepted hierarchy-of-controls model. The discussion could include comments on how widely products have been used or programs implemented. The qualitative discussion should be specific as to the various products developed by the program and the extent of their use by specific entities (industry, labor, government, and so on) for specific purposes. Whether the products have resulted in changes in the workplace or in the reduction of risk should be discussed. The recognition accorded to the program or the facilities by its peers (such as recognition as a "center of excellence" by national and international communities) should be considered in the assessment. To be highly ranked, a program should have high performance in most of the relevant questions in this section. An aspect of the evaluation can be whether the same changes in stakeholder activities and behaviors would probably have occurred without NIOSH efforts.

III.B.8. Review of End Outcomes
(Figure 2, Box F)

It is necessary for the EC to assess, to the greatest extent possible, NIOSH's contribution to end outcomes—improvements in workplace health and safety (impact). For purposes of this evaluation, end outcomes are health-related changes that are a result of program activities, including decreases in injuries, illnesses, deaths and exposures or risk. Data on reductions in work-related injuries, illnesses, and hazardous exposures will be available for some programs, and in some cases they will be quantifiable. It is possible, however, to evaluate the impact of a NIOSH research program using either intermediate outcomes or end outcomes. If there is no direct evidence of improvements in health and safety, intermediate outcomes may be used as proxies for end outcomes in assessing impact as long as the EC qualifies its findings. The EC will describe the realized or potential benefits of the NIOSH program. Examples of realized intermediate outcomes are new regulations and widely accepted guidelines, work practices, and procedures, all of which may contribute measurably to enhancing health and safety in the workplace.

The FC recognizes that assessing the causal relationship between NIOSH research and specific occupational health and safety outcomes is a major challenge because NIOSH does not have direct responsibility or authority for implementing its research findings in the workplace. Furthermore, the benefits of NIOSH research program outputs can be realized, potential, or limited to the knowledge gained. Studies that conclude with negative results may nevertheless have incorporated excellent science and contribute to the knowledge base. The generation of important knowledge is a recognized form of outcome in the absence of measurable impacts.

The impact of an outcome depends on the existence of a "receptor" for research results, such as a regulatory agency, a professional organization, an employer, and an employee organization. The EC should consider questions related to the various stages that lead to outputs, such as these:

1. Did NIOSH research identify a gap in protection or a means of reducing risk?
2. Did NIOSH convey that information to potential users in a usable form?
3. Were NIOSH research results (for example, recommendations, technologies) applied?
4. Did the applied results lead to desired outcomes?

Quantitative data are preferable to qualitative, but qualitative analysis may be necessary. Sources of quantitative data include the following:

- Bureau of Labor Statistics (BLS) data on fatal occupational injuries (the Census of Fatal Occupational Injuries) and nonfatal occupational injuries and illnesses (the annual Survey of Occupational Injury and Illnesses)
- NIOSH intramural surveillance systems, such as the National Electronic Injury Surveillance System, the coal-worker x-ray surveillance program, and agricultural-worker surveys conducted by NIOSH in collaboration with USDA
- State-based surveillance systems, such as the NIOSH-funded ABLES, and the SENSOR programs (for asthma, pesticides, silicosis, noise-induced hearing loss, dermatitis, and burns)
- Selected state worker-compensation programs
- Exposure data collected in the OSHA Integrated Management Information System

The FC is unaware of mechanisms for surveillance of many occupationally related chronic illnesses, such as cancers that arise from long exposure to chemicals and other stressors. The incidence and prevalence of many such outcomes are best evaluated by investigator-initiated research. Research that leads to new, effective surveillance concepts or programs warrants special recognition.

The EC should recognize the strengths and weaknesses of outcome data sources. Quantitative accident, injury, illness, and employment data and databases are subject to error and bias and should be used by the EC only for drawing inferences after critical evaluation and examination of available corroborating data. For example, it is widely recognized that occupational illnesses are poorly documented in the BLS Survey of Occupational Injuries and Illnesses, which captures only incident cases among active workers. It is difficult for health practitioners to diagnose work-relatedness of most illnesses that may not be exclusively related to work; furthermore, few practitioners are adequately trained to make such an assessment. Many of those illnesses have long latencies and do not appear until years after people have left the employment in question. Surveillance programs may systematically undercount some categories of workers, such as contingent workers.

In addition to measures of illness and injury, measures of exposure to chemical and physical agents and to safety and ergonomic hazards can be useful. Exposure or probability of exposure can serve as an appropriate proxy for disease or injury when a well-described occupational exposure-health association exists. In such instances, a decrease in exposure can be accepted as evidence that the end outcome of reduced illness or injury is being achieved. That is necessary particularly when the latent period between exposure and disease outcome, as in the case of asbestos exposure and lung cancer, makes effective evaluation of the relevant end outcome infeasible.

As an example of how an exposure level can serve as a proxy, reduction in the number of sites that exceed an OSHA PEL or an American Conference of Governmental Industrial Hygienists threshold limit value is a quantitative measure of improvement of occupational health awareness and reduction of risk. In addition to exposure level, the number of people exposed and the distribution of exposure levels are important. Those data are available from multiple databases and studies of exposure. Apart from air monitoring, such measures of exposure as biohazard controls, reduction in requirements for use of personal protective equipment, and reduction in ergonomic risks are important.

Challenges posed by inadequate or inaccurate measurement systems should not drive programs out of difficult fields of study, and the EC will need to be aware of such a possibility. In particular, contingent and informal working arrangements that place workers at greatest risk are also those on which surveillance information is almost totally lacking, so novel methods for measuring impact may be required.

The commitment of industry, labor, and government to health and safety are critical external factors. Several measures of that commitment can be useful for the EC: monetary commitments, attitude, staffing, and surveys of relative importance. To the extent that resources allocated to safety and health are limiting factors, the EC should explicitly assess NIOSH performance in the context of constraints.

Questions to Guide the Evaluation Committee

1. What are the amounts and qualities of relevant end-outcomes data (such as injuries, illness, exposure, and productivity affected by health)?
2. What are the temporal trends in those data?
3. Is there objective evidence of improvement in occupational safety or health?

4. To what degree is the NIOSH program or subprogram responsible for improvement in occupational safety or health?
5. If there is no time trend in the data, how do findings compare with data from other comparable US groups or the corresponding populations in other countries?
6. What is the evidence that external factors have affected outcomes or outcome measures?
7. Has the program been responsible for outcomes outside the United States that have not been described in another category?

Assessment

The EC should provide a qualitative assessment of the program and subprogram impact, discussing the evidence of reductions in injuries and illnesses or their appropriate proxies.

III.B.9. Review of Potential Outcomes

There may be health and safety impacts not yet appreciated and other beneficial social, economic, and environmental outcomes as a result of NIOSH activities. NIOSH study results may be influential outside the United States, and there may be evidence of implementation of NIOSH recommendations and training programs abroad.

Questions to Guide the Evaluation Committee

1. Is the program likely to produce a favorable change that has not yet occurred or not been appreciated?
2. Has the program been responsible for social, economic, security, or environmental outcomes?
3. Has the program's work had an impact on occupational health and safety in other countries?

Assessment

The EC may discuss other outcomes, including beneficial changes that have not yet occurred; social, economic, security, or environmental outcomes; and the impact that NIOSH has had on international occupational safety and health.

III.B.10. Summary Evaluation Ratings and Rationale

The EC should use its expert judgment to rate the relevance and impact of the overall research program by first summarizing its assessments of the major subprograms and then appropriately weighting the subprograms to determine the overall program ratings.

Table 5 provides some background context to aid the EC in reaching overall ratings for relevance and impact. The EC could consider the items in Table 5 for each subprogram then for the overall program and assess the relevance of the research subprograms and program by reviewing earlier responses to the questions in Sections III.B.2 through III.B.5 (reviews of program challenges, strategic goals and objectives, inputs, and activities). Items 1-4 in Table 5 are pertinent to assessing relevance.

To assess overall impact, the EC first needs to consider the available evidence of changes in work-related risks and adverse effects and external factors related to the changes. The EC should review the responses to the questions in Sections III.B.6 through III.B.8 (reviews of outputs, intermediate outcomes, and end outcomes) and systematically assess the impact of the research program and its subprograms. Items 5-7 in Table 5 will be helpful. The EC should evaluate separately the impact of the research and the impact of transfer activities. Transfer activities occur in two contexts: NIOSH efforts to translate intellectual products into practice and stakeholder efforts to integrate NIOSH results into the workplace. High impact assessments require the EC's judgment that the research program has contributed to outcomes; for example, outcomes have occurred earlier than they would have or are better than they would have been in the absence of the research program,

TABLE 5 Background Context for Program Relevance and Impact

Assess the following for each subprogram:

1. Relevance of current and recently completed research and transfer activities to objective improvements in workplace safety and health.
2. Contributions of NIOSH research and transfer activities to changes in work-related practices and reduction in workplace exposures, illnesses, or injuries.
3. Contributions of NIOSH research and transfer activities to improvements in work-related practices.
4. Contributions of NIOSH research to productivity, security, or environmental quality (beneficial side effects).
5. Evidence of reduction of risk in the workplace (intermediate outcome).
6. Evidence of reduction in workplace exposure, illness, or injuries (end outcome).
7. Evidence of external factors that prevented translation of NIOSH research results into intermediate or end outcomes.

or outcomes would have occurred were it not for external factors beyond NIOSH's control or ability to plan around.

The EC must assign one overall integer score for the *relevance* of the research program to the improvement of occupational safety and health and one overall integer score for the *impact* of the program on the improvement of occupational safety and health. The EC will use its expert judgment, summary assessment of research-program elements, and any appropriate information to arrive at those two scores. In light of substantial differences among the types of research programs that will be reviewed and the challenge to arrive at a summative evaluation of both relevance and impact, the FC chose not to construct an algorithm to produce the two final ratings.

Relevance and impact scores will be based on five-point categorical scales established by the FC (see Boxes 2 and 3) in which 1 is the lowest and 5 the highest rating. The FC has made an effort to establish mutually exclusive rating categories in the scales. When the basis of a rating fits more than one category, the highest applicable score should be assigned. It is up to the EC to determine how individual subprograms should influence final scores. Single integer values should be assigned. Final program ratings will consist of integer scores for relevance and impact and prose justification of the scores.

Box 2 includes the criteria for scoring the overall relevance of the NIOSH research program. As discussed in previous sections, numerous factors can be considered in assessing relevance. The scoring criteria focus on two: the EC assessment

---

BOX 2
Scoring Criteria for Relevance

5 = Research is in high-priority subject areas and NIOSH is significantly engaged in appropriate transfer activities for completed research projects/reported research results.
4 = Research is in priority subject areas and NIOSH is engaged in appropriate transfer activities for completed research projects/reported research results.
3 = Research is in high priority or priority subject areas, but NIOSH is not engaged in appropriate transfer activities; or research focuses on lesser priorities but NIOSH is engaged in appropriate transfer activities.
2 = Research program is focused on lesser priorities and NIOSH is not engaged in or planning some appropriate transfer activities.
1 = Research program is not focused on priorities and NIOSH is not engaged in transfer activities.

> **BOX 3**
> **Scoring Criteria for Impact**
>
> 5 = Research program has made major contribution(s) to worker health and safety on the basis of end outcomes or well-accepted intermediate outcomes.
> 4 = Research program has made some contributions to end outcomes or well-accepted intermediate outcomes.
> 3 = Research program activities are ongoing and outputs are produced that are likely to result in improvements in worker health and safety (with explanation of why not rated higher). Well accepted outcomes have not been recorded.
> 2 = Research program activities are ongoing and outputs are produced that may result in new knowledge or technology, but only limited application is expected. Well accepted outcomes have not been recorded.
> 1 = Research activities and outputs do not result in or are NOT likely to have any application.

of whether the program appropriately sets priorities among research needs and the EC assessment of how engaged the program is in appropriate transfer activities. Table 6 provides some guidance regarding how the EC may weight research priorities and transfer levels when determining relevance scores.

The EC will consider both completed research and research that is in progress and related to likely future improvements in its assessment of relevance. The EC should keep in mind how well the program has considered the frequency and severity of the problems being addressed; whether appropriate attention has been directed to both sexes, vulnerable populations, or hard-to-reach workplaces; and whether the different needs of large and small businesses have been accounted for. It is up to the EC to determine how to consider external factors in assigning program scores.

Box 3 includes the criteria established for the rating of impact. In general, the EC will consider completed research outputs during the assessment of impact. In assigning a score for impact, it is important to recognize that a "major contribution" (required for a score of 5) does not imply that the NIOSH program was solely responsible for observed improvements in worker health and safety. Many factors may be required to effect improvements. The EC could say that NIOSH made "major contributions" if the improvements would not have occurred when they did without NIOSH efforts.

TABLE 6 Guidance for Weighting Research Priority and Engagement in Appropriate Transfer Activities in the Application of Relevance Score

Assessment of Research Priority	Engagement in Applicable Transfer Activities	Applicable Score
High priority	Significantly engaged	5
High priority	Engaged	4
High priority	Not engaged	3
Priority	Significantly engaged	4
Priority	Engaged	4
Priority	Not engaged	3
Lesser priority	Significantly engaged	3
Lesser priority	Engaged	3
Lesser priority	Not engaged	2
Not focused on priorities	Significantly engaged	2
Not focused on priorities	Engaged	2
Not focused on priorities	Not engaged	1

The FC has some concern that the imposed scoring criteria for impact might be considered a promotion of the conventional occupational-health research paradigm that focuses on health-effects and technology research without much emphasis on the socioeconomic, policy, surveillance, and diffusion research (as opposed to diffusion activities) needed to effect change. The EC should remember that not all intermediate outcomes occur in the workplace. Important outcomes that NIOSH can effect also occur much farther out on the causal chain. NIOSH, for example, has an important role to play in generating knowledge that may contribute to changing norms in the insurance industry, in health-care practice, in public-health practice, and in the community at large. The EC may find that some of those issues need to be addressed and considered as external factors that facilitate or limit application of more traditional research findings. Given the rapidly changing nature of work and the workforce and some of the intractable problems in manufacturing, mining, and some other fields, the EC is encouraged to think beyond the traditional paradigm.

III.C. Assessment of NIOSH Process for Targeting Priority Research Needs and Committee Assessment of Emerging Issues

The second charge to the EC is the assessment of the research program's effectiveness in targeting new research and identifying emerging issues in occupational safety and health most relevant to future improvements in workplace protection. The EC is also asked to provide a qualitative narrative assessment of the program's efforts and to make suggestions about emerging issues that the program should be prepared to address. Among the most challenging aspects of research in illness and injury prevention are the identification of new or emerging needs or trends and the formulation of a research response that appropriately uses scarce resources in anticipation of them.

The EC should review the procedures that NIOSH and the research program have in place to identify needed research relevant to the NIOSH mission and should review the success that NIOSH has had in identifying and addressing research related to emerging issues. It should examine leading indicators from appropriate federal agencies, such as EPA, the Department of Labor, the National Institute of Standards and Technology, NIH, DOD, and the Department of Commerce. Those indicators should track new technologies, new products, new processes, and disease or injury trends.

One source of information deserving particular attention is NIOSH HHE reports. The HHE program offers a potential mechanism for identifying emerging research needs that could be incorporated as input into each of the programs evaluated. The EC should determine whether the program under review appropriately considers pertinent HHE investigation findings. Additional emerging issues may be revealed through consideration of NIOSH and the NIOSH-funded FACE reports, the AOEC reports, the US Chemical Safety Board investigations, and SENSOR and other state-based surveillance programs. Appropriate federal advisory committees and other stakeholder groups should also be consulted to provide qualitative information.

The EC should systematically assess how the research program and its subprograms target new research by evaluating each subprogram for the items listed in Table 7. The EC will have to determine how best to weight subprogram contributions in the program's targeting of new research.

TABLE 7 Targeting of New Research and Identification of Emerging Issues

Assess the following for each subprogram:

1. Past and present effectiveness in targeting most relevant research needs.
2. Effectiveness in targeting research in fields most relevant to future improvements in occupational safety and health.
3. Contribution of NIOSH research to enhancement of capacity in government or other research institutions.

Questions to Guide the Evaluation Committee

1. What information does NIOSH review to identify emerging research needs?
   a. What is the process for review?
   b. How often does the process take place?
   c. How are NIOSH staff scientists and NIOSH leadership engaged?
   d. What is the process for moving from ideas to formal planning and resource allocation?
2. How are stakeholders involved?
   a. What advisory or stakeholder groups are asked to identify emerging research targets?
   b. How often are such groups consulted, and how are suggestions followed up?
3. What new research targets have been identified for future development in the program under evaluation?
   a. How were they identified?
   b. Were lessons that could help to identify other emerging issues learned?
   c. Does the EC agree with the issues identified and selected as important and with the NIOSH response, or were important issues overlooked?
   d. Is there evidence of unwise expenditure of resources on unimportant issues?

The EC members should use their expert judgment both to evaluate the emerging research targets identified by NIOSH and to provide recommendations to NIOSH regarding additional research that NIOSH has not yet identified. Recommendations should include a brief statement of their rationale.

IV. EVALUATION COMMITTEE REPORT TEMPLATE

Consistency and comparability among EC report formats is desirable, but the FC recognizes that each NIOSH research program is different and that each EC is independent. The outline provided in Box 4 flows from the FC's review of NIOSH's generalized logic model (Figure 1), the evaluation flowchart (Figure 2), and the assessment model described earlier in this document. The EC should feel free to use or adapt this outline as necessary when organizing its final report. The FC encourages each EC to look at prior EC reports for organizational ideas.

BOX 4
Suggested Outline for Evaluation Committee Reports

I. Introduction
This section should be a brief descriptive summary of the history of the program (and subprograms) being evaluated with respect to pre-NORA, NORA 1, and current and future plans of the research program presented by NIOSH. It should present the context for the research on safety and health; goals, objectives, and resources; groupings of subprograms; and any other important pertinent information. (A list of the NIOSH materials reviewed should be provided in Appendix C.)

II. Evaluation of Programs and Subprograms (Charge 1)
A. Evaluation summary (should include a brief summary of the evaluation with respect to impact and relevance, scores for impact and relevance, and summary statements).
B. Strategic goals and objectives: should describe assessment of the program and sub-programs for relevance.
C. Review of inputs: should describe adequacy of inputs to achieve goals.
D. Review of activities: should describe assessment of the relevance of the activities.
E. Review of research-program outputs: should describe assessment of relevance and potential usefulness of the research program.
F. Review of intermediate outcomes and causal impact: should describe assessment of the intermediate outcomes and the attribution to NIOSH; should include the likely impacts and recent outcomes in the assessment.
G. Review of end outcomes: should describe the end outcomes related to health and safety and provides an assessment of the type and degree of attribution to NIOSH.
H. Review of other outcomes: should discuss health and safety impacts that have not yet occurred; beneficial social, economic, and environmental outcomes; and international dimensions and outcomes.
I. Summary of ratings and rationale.

III. NIOSH Targeting of New Research and Identification of Emerging Issues (Charge 2)
The EC should assess the progress that the NIOSH program has made in targeting new research in occupational safety and health. The EC should assess whether the NIOSH program has identified important emerging issues that appear especially important in terms of relevance to the mission of NIOSH. The EC should respond to NIOSH's perspective and add its own recommendations.

IV. Recommendations for Program Improvement
On the basis of the review and evaluation of the program, the EC may provide recommendations for improving the relevance of the NIOSH research program to health and safety conditions in the workplace and the impact of the research program on health and safety in the workplace.

Appendix A — Framework Document
Appendix B — Methods and Information-Gathering
Appendix C — List of **NIOSH** and Related Materials Collected in the Process of the Evaluation

B

Methods: Committee Information Gathering

This appendix provides additional detail regarding the methods used by the Institute of Medicine (IOM) Committee to Review the National Institute for Occupational Safety and Health (NIOSH) Personal Protective Technology (PPT) Program to gather information to carry out its work.

COMMITTEE MEETINGS

The committee held three meetings during the course of this study. The first two meetings included open sessions for information gathering. The agendas for these open sessions appear below. The third meeting was held in closed session. The committee also participated in a site visit at the NIOSH facility in Bruceton, Pennsylvania (agenda below).

APPENDIX B

MEETING 1
September 28, 2007
Committee to Review the NIOSH Personal Protective Technology Program
The National Academies Keck Center
500 Fifth Street, N.W.
Washington, D.C.

AGENDA

OPEN SESSION

8:00 a.m.   Welcome and Introductions
            John Gallagher, Chair

8:15   Charge to the Committee-NIOSH Overview
            Lewis Wade, NIOSH Senior Science Advisor

8:45   Overview and Scope of the PPT Program
            Les Boord, Director, National Personal Protective Technology Laboratory (NPPTL) (*PPT Program Manager*)

            Overview and Scope of the PPT Program
            Maryann D'Alessandro, Associate Director for Science, NPPTL (*PPT Program Coordinator*)

            Discussion

9:45   Break

10:00   PPT Presentations—Reduce Exposure to Inhalation Hazards

            - Respirator Certification (SG 1, Obj 1)
              Les Boord, Director, NPPTL
            - CBRN (chemical, biological, radiological, and nuclear) Respirator Standards (SG 1, Obj 2)
              Jon Szalajda, Branch Chief, Policy and Standards
            - Mine Escape Respirators (SG 1, Obj 3)
              Les Boord, Director, NPPTL
            - Anthropometrics and Fit (SG 1, Obj 4)
              Roland Berry Ann, Deputy Director, NPPTL

Discussion

- Pandemic Preparedness (SG 1, Obj 5)
  Roland Berry Ann, Deputy Director, NPPTL
  Ron Shaffer, Branch Chief, Technology Research
- Nanotechnology (SG 1, Obj 6)
  Ron Shaffer, Branch Chief, Technology Research
- End-of-Service-Life Indicators (SG 1, Obj 7)
  Ron Shaffer, Branch Chief, Technology Research
- Surveillance (SG 1, Obj 8)
  Maryann D'Alessandro, Associate Director for Science, NPPTL

Discussion

11:45   Lunch

12:15 p.m.   PPT Presentations—Reduce Exposure to Injury Hazards

- Warning Devices for Fire Services (SG 3, Obj 1)
  Bill Haskell, Physical Scientist, NPPTL

1:00   PPT Presentations—Reduce Exposure to Dermal Hazards

- Chemical Dermal Hazards (SG 2, Obj 1)
  Ron Shaffer, Branch Chief, Technology Research
- Emergency Responder Protective Clothing (SG 2, Obj 2)
  Physiological and Ergonomic Impact (SG 2, Obj 3)
  Bill Haskell, Physical Scientist, NPPTL

Discussion

2:00   Wrap-up and Discussion
       Les Boord and Maryann D'Alessandro

2:30   Adjourn Open Session

APPENDIX B

SITE VISIT

November 8, 2007
Committee to Review the NIOSH Personal Protective Technology Program

National Personal Protective Technology Laboratory
Cochrans Mill Road, Pittsburgh, Pa.

AGENDA

OPEN SESSION

Breakfast at the Hotel

7:00 a.m.	Board Shuttle
7:15	Shuttle Departure—Hotel to NPPTL Facility
8:30	Tours of Labs
12:00 p.m.	Lunch
12:30	Continue Lab Tours
2:30	Adjourn

MEETING 2

December 17, 2007
Committee to Review the NIOSH Personal Protective Technology Program
The National Academies Keck Center
500 Fifth Street, N.W.
Washington, D.C.

AGENDA

OPEN SESSION

8:00 a.m.   Welcome
                John Gallagher, Chair

8:05   Discussions with NIOSH staff

           Questions to NIOSH staff

- Extramural research
  What is the current role of the PPT intramural program in identifying or setting the topics for extramural research requests? Description of the relationship between NPPTL activities and NIOSH extramural research program.

- Priority setting in the intramural program
  Could you provide more details on the process? How long has that process been in place?

- Training
  What do you see as the role of the PPT program in training and education regarding the use of PPE? What current efforts focus on training issues?

- Rule making
  Modular approach to rule making—what is under way, what is planned?
  What are the normal time frame and process for rule making—general overview?
  How did the CBRN process differ in timing or mechanics?

- Post-certification efforts
  Could you provide more information on product and facility audits? Who does the audits and how often? How are products selected for the audits?

9:45 Break

PANEL DISCUSSIONS

Questions to the Panelists

1. What recent improvements in personal protective technology have led to documented decreases in hazardous exposures, morbidity, or mortality in the workplace? In what ways and to what degree has the NIOSH PPT program played a role in those improvements?

   - Please identify those items where the PPT Program's work is especially relevant and also efforts that are less relevant to its mission.
   - Please give specific examples of NIOSH's success and impact in this area and examples where there are opportunities to make a greater impact.

2. What do you see as significant *emerging* research needs or opportunities in PPT? How does NIOSH obtain stakeholder input into identifying these emerging issues and targeting new research?
3. What NIOSH products or services do you use and what ideas do you have for improving these products or services?
4. What could the NIOSH PPT program be doing that it is not now doing with respect to research, policy and standards development, and respirator certification? What should the program continue to do in these areas?

10:00   Panel 1: Federal and State Agencies

   Moderator: *Howard Cohen*

   Panelists:
   John Steelnack, Occupational Safety and Health Administration (OSHA)
   Stephan Graham, InterAgency Board for Equipment Standardization and Interoperability (IAB)
   David Caretti, Department of Defense
   Laura McMullen and Jeff Kravitz, Mine Safety and Health Administration (MSHA)

   Discussion

11:00   Panel 2: Employers and Employees

   Moderator: *Knut Ringen*

   Panelists:
   Dee Woodhull, ORC International
   Dean Cox, Fairfax County Fire Department
   Dennis O'Dell, United Mine Workers Association (invited)
   Robert Glenn, National Industrial Sand Association

   Discussion

12:15 p.m.   Lunch

1:00   Panel 3: PPT Manufacturers

   Moderator: *Janice Bradley*

   Panelists:
   James Zeigler, DuPont
   Zane Frund, Mine Safety Appliances (MSA)
   Rob Freese, Globe Manufacturing
   Craig Colton, 3M

   Discussion

APPENDIX B

2:15 Panel 4: Standard Setting and Certifying Organizations

        Moderator: *Jimmy Perkins*

        Panelists:
        Jeff Stull, International Personnel Protection, ASTM International
        Bruce Teele, National Fire Protection Association
        Pat Gleason, Safety Equipment Institute

        Discussion

3:15 Break

3:45 Discussions with NIOSH Staff

5:00 Public Comment (registered speakers)

5:45 Adjourn

Stakeholder Respondents

The following individuals responded to the committee's invitation for comments on the NIOSH Personal Protective Technology Program:

Don Aldridge
Lion Apparel

Rick Avila
Marriott's Maui Ocean Club

JoAnn J. Bowman
Lake Region Hospital

Lisa Brosseau
University of Minnesota

Sue Champagne
Maricopa Integrated Health System

Alan Hack
Independent Consultant

Don Hewitt
Terrorism Research Center

Frank Lafferty, Jr.
Haddon Heights Fire Department, New Jersey

Dennis Ottney
SafetyTech International, Inc.

C

Information Provided by the NIOSH PPT Program

Some of the materials are available online at the following NIOSH website: http://www.cdc.gov/niosh/nas/ppt. All of the materials are available for review at the National Academies through the study's public access file.

Gao, P., and B. Tomasovic. 2005. Change in tensile properties of neoprene and nitrile gloves after repeated exposures to acetone and thermal decontamination. *Journal of Occupational and Environmental Hygiene* 2:543-552.

Gao, P., N. El-Ayouby, and J. T. Wassell. 2005. Change in permeation parameters and the decontamination efficacy of three chemical protective gloves after repeated exposures to solvents and thermal decontaminations. *American Journal of Industrial Medicine* 47:131-143.

Gao, P., W. King, and R. Shaffer. 2007. Review of chamber design requirements for testing of personal protective clothing ensembles. *Journal of Occupational and Environmental Hygiene* 4:562-571.

NIOSH. 2006. *Personal Protective Technology Program quad charts 2006.* Distributed to the Committee to Review the NIOSH Personal Protective Technology Program, September 28, 2007.

NIOSH. 2007. *Wrap-up presentation of the Personal Protective Technology Program.* Presentation to the Committee to Review the NIOSH Personal Protective Technology Program, September 28, 2007.

NIOSH. 2007. *Evidence for the Personal Protective Technology Program.* Presentation to the Committee to Review the NIOSH Personal Protective Technology Program, September 28, 2007.

NIOSH. 2007. *Evidence package for the Committee to Review the NIOSH Personal Protective Technology Program,* September 14, 2007.

NIOSH. 2007. *Personal Protective Technology Program quad charts 2007.* Distributed to the Committee to Review the NIOSH Personal Protective Technology Program, September 28, 2007.

NIOSH. 2007. *PPT Program response to IOM questions.* Distributed to the Committee to Review the NIOSH Personal Protective Technology Program, October 19, 2007.

NIOSH. No date. *Development of colorimetric indicators: A new technique to determine acid, base, and aldehyde contaminations.* Distributed to the Committee to Review the NIOSH Personal Protective Technology Program, November 8, 2007.

NIOSH. 2007. *Summary of renovation costs.* Distributed to the Committee to Review the NIOSH Personal Protective Technology Program, November 8, 2007.
NIOSH. 2007. *Permeation Calculator (Version 2.4) Software.* Distributed to the Committee to Review the NIOSH Personal Protective Technology Program, November 8, 2007.
NIOSH. 2007. *TSI Fractional Efficiency Filter Test: Fractional penetration.* Distributed to the Committee to Review the NIOSH Personal Protective Technology Program, November 8, 2007.
NIOSH. 2007. *PPT Program response to questions to NIOSH: Working Group 1.* Distributed to the Committee to Review the NIOSH Personal Protective Technology Program, November 14, 2007.
NIOSH. 2007. *PPT Program response to questions to NIOSH: Working Group 3.* Distributed to the Committee to Review the NIOSH Personal Protective Technology Program, November 14, 2007.
NIOSH. 2007. *PPT Program response to questions to NIOSH: Working Group 2.* Distributed to the Committee to Review the NIOSH Personal Protective Technology Program, December 10, 2007.
NIOSH. 2007. *PPT response to 12/06/07 teleconference: ESLI test procedure inquiry.* Distributed to the Committee to Review the NIOSH Personal Protective Technology Program, December 13, 2007.
NIOSH. 2007. *PPT response to inquiry regarding respirator certification numbers.* Distributed to the Committee to Review the NIOSH Personal Protective Technology Program, December 13, 2007.
NIOSH. 2007. *PPT training vision.* Distributed to the Committee to Review the NIOSH Personal Protective Technology Program, December 13, 2007.
NIOSH. No date. *FY03 processing data for air-purifying respirator applications.* Distributed to the Committee to Review the NIOSH Personal Protective Technology Program, December 14, 2007.
NIOSH. 2007. *FY03 processing data for air-supplied respirator applications.* Distributed to the Committee to Review the NIOSH Personal Protective Technology Program, December 14, 2007.
NIOSH. 2007. *FY04 processing data for air-purifying respirator applications.* Distributed to the Committee to Review the NIOSH Personal Protective Technology Program, December 14, 2007.
NIOSH. 2007. *FY04 processing data for air-supplied respirator applications.* NIOSH. Distributed to the Committee to Review the NIOSH Personal Protective Technology Program, December 14, 2007.
NIOSH. 2007. *FY05 processing data for air-purifying respirator applications.* Distributed to the Committee to Review the NIOSH Personal Protective Technology Program, December 14, 2007.
NIOSH. 2007. *FY05 processing data for air-supplied respirator applications.* Distributed to the Committee to Review the NIOSH Personal Protective Technology Program, December 14, 2007.
NIOSH. 2007. *FY06 processing data for air-purifying respirator applications.* Distributed to the Committee to Review the NIOSH Personal Protective Technology Program, December 14, 2007.
NIOSH. 2007. *FY06 processing data for air-supplied respirator applications.* Distributed to the Committee to Review the NIOSH Personal Protective Technology Program, December 14, 2007.
NIOSH. 2007. *FY07 processing data for air-purifying respirator applications.* Distributed to the Committee to Review the NIOSH Personal Protective Technology Program, December 14, 2007.
NIOSH. 2007. *FY07 processing data for air-supplied respirator applications.* Distributed to the Committee to Review the NIOSH Personal Protective Technology Program, December 14, 2007.
NIOSH. 2008. *PPT Program FTE Summary.* Submitted to the Committee to Review the NIOSH Personal Protective Technology Program, February 8, 2008.
NIOSH. 2008. *PPT Program response to questions to NIOSH dated 01-04-08.* Submitted to the Committee to Review the NIOSH Personal Protective Technology Program, February 8, 2008.
NIOSH. 2008. *National Personal Protective Technology Laboratory Strategic Plan FY2008.* Submitted to the Committee to Review the NIOSH Personal Protective Technology Program, February 8, 2008.
Zhuang, Z., and B. Bradtmiller. 2005. Head-and-face anthropometric survey of U.S. respirator uses. *Journal of Occupational and Environmental Hygiene* 2:567-576.

D

Biographical Sketches of Committee Members

E. JOHN GALLAGHER, M.D. (*Chair*), is university chair of the department of emergency medicine at Albert Einstein College of Medicine and Montefiore Medical Center where he serves as a professor in the departments of emergency medicine, medicine, and epidemiology and population health. Dr. Gallagher's research targets out-of-hospital cardiac arrest, measurement and management of acute pain, and diagnostic testing and reasoning. For more than 30 years, he has focused on strategies to optimize care of the medically underserved inner-city population of the Bronx. Dr. Gallagher received his medical degree from the University of Pennsylvania School of Medicine in 1972. His service to professional organizations includes serving as president of the Association of Academic Chairs of Emergency Medicine and as editor of several medical journals. He has published numerous peer-reviewed articles and book chapters on a wide range of emergency medicine topics. Dr. Gallagher served on the Institute of Medicine (IOM) Committee for Developing Reusable Facemasks for Use During an Influenza Pandemic, as a consultant to the IOM Committee on Increasing Rates of Organ Donation, and as a reviewer for the IOM report *Hospital-Based Emergency Care: At the Breaking Point*. Dr. Gallagher was elected a member of the IOM in 2002.

ROGER L. BARKER, Ph.D., is the Burlington Distinguished Professor in the department of textile engineering, chemistry, and science at North Carolina State University and director of the Center for Research on Textile Protection and

Comfort. He has been engaged in research and standards development for protective clothing for more than 20 years and is internationally recognized for his work in the field of protective clothing systems. Dr. Barker has published many technical papers on the protective properties of textile materials and clothing and on testing methods used for evaluation. He is active in the National Fire Protection Association (NFPA), ASTM International, and the International Organization for Standardization (ISO) committees involved in the development of standards for measurement for personal protective equipment. Dr. Barker holds B.S. and M.S. degrees in physics from the University of Tennessee and a Ph.D. in textile and polymer science from Clemson University.

HOWARD J. COHEN, Ph.D., is a professor and chair of the occupational safety and health department at the University of New Haven. He formerly was the manager of industrial hygiene at the Olin Corporation and editor-in-chief of the *American Industrial Hygiene Association (AIHA) Journal*. He is a graduate of Boston University where he received a B.A. degree in biology. Dr. Cohen received his master of public health and doctorate of philosophy degrees in industrial health from the University of Michigan. He is certified in the comprehensive practice of industrial hygiene (CIH) by the American Board of Industrial Hygiene. Dr. Cohen is the former chair of the American National Standards Institute (ANSI) Z88.2 committee on respiratory protection and a current member of the editorial board of the *Journal of Occupational and Environmental Hygiene*. He is the past chair of the AIHA's respiratory protection committee, a past president of the Connecticut River Valley Chapter of the American Industrial Hygiene Association, and a past officer and treasurer of the American Board of Industrial Hygiene.

JANICE COMER-BRADLEY, M.A., is technical director of the International Safety Equipment Association (ISEA), where she directs the voluntary standards-setting activities of 13 product groups representing suppliers of safety and health equipment. She works closely with federal regulatory agencies and outside standards bodies to influence activities that affect the manufacture, use, and distribution of safety equipment, and she represents ISEA on numerous standards committee and government panels. Ms. Bradley earned a B.S. degree from the University of Dayton and a master's degree in environmental studies from Brown University. Ms. Bradley has spent her entire career in the safety and health field. Prior to her work at ISEA she was the director of environmental health and safety for the Rockefeller University in New York City, the university health and safety officer for Brown University, and the safety specialist for the Department of Veterans Affairs Medical Center in Dayton, Ohio. Ms. Bradley is a certified safety professional by the American Society of Safety Engineers and an adjunct professor at Georgetown University where she teaches a graduate-level course in the M.B.A. program that introduces future business leaders to workplace safety and health issues. She served on the National Research Council (NRC) Committee on the Review of the NIOSH-BLS Respirator Use Survey Program.

ELIZABETH A. CORLEY, Ph.D., is assistant professor in the School of Public Affairs at Arizona State University. She is also an affiliated faculty member in the Consortium for Science, Policy, and Outcomes (CSPO) and the School of Sustainability at Arizona State University. Dr. Corley's current research is focused on the areas of evaluation and science policy. Her funded research projects focus on the development of innovative methodologies for program evaluation, the evaluation of science and engineering research centers, and the social impacts of science. Dr. Corley is currently principal investigator for the external evaluation of the Learning in Formal and Informal Environments Center funded by the National Science Foundation (NSF) and serves as a co-principal investigator for the NSF-funded Center for Nanotechnology in Society at Arizona State University (CNS-ASU). She currently serves as a member of the editorial board for *Research Evaluation*. Prior to joining ASU in 2003, Dr. Corley held teaching and research positions at Columbia University, Georgia Institute of Technology, and Bucknell University. While attending the Georgia Institute of Technology, she earned three degrees in civil engineering and a Ph.D. in public policy.

RICHARD M. DUFFY, M.Sc., has been involved with worker occupational health and safety issues for more than 30 years, the past 29 years at the International Association of Fire Fighters (IAFF), where he is assistant to the general president, responsible for the IAFF's activities addressing occupational medicine, safety, and health. He has been involved in numerous committees involving firefighters' and other workers' safety and health, including those of the federal government, state governments, NFPA, ANSI, and ISO. He has been actively involved in addressing protective clothing and equipment for workers. He served as chairman of the NFPA Technical Correlating Committee for Fire and Emergency Services Protective Clothing and Equipment. He directed the National Aeronautics and Space Administration-Federal Emergency Management Agency program Project FIRES (Firefighters Integrated Response Equipment System), which under the auspices of the IAFF continues to work toward the development of state-of-the-art protective clothing and equipment, including the management of the new IAFF initiative Project HEROES (Homeland Emergency Response Operational and Equipment Systems). Mr. Duffy is responsible for the coordination and technical aspects of the IAFF-IAFC (International Association of Fire Chiefs) Joint Wellness-Fitness Initiative for Fire Fighters, including the Wellness-Fitness Program, and has been directly responsible for IAFF efforts in addressing infectious diseases, including pandemic flu and proper recommendations for personal protective equipment. He has served as a member on the NRC Panel for Fire Research. Mr. Duffy holds bachelor of science degrees in environmental health and in business management and a master of science degree in occupational and environmental health sciences.

JAMES S. JOHNSON, Ph.D., C.I.H., QEP, has worked at the Lawrence Livermore National Laboratory (LLNL) since 1972. His position from November 2000 was section leader of the Chemical and Biological Safety Section of the Safety Programs Division. Throughout his career at LLNL, Dr. Johnson was involved with respiratory protection and personal protective equipment as the respiratory program administrator, research scientist, and division and section manager. He is an AIHA fellow; a member of the NFPA Technical Correlating Committee on Fire and Emergency Services Protective Clothing and Equipment; a member of the NFPA Respiratory Protection Equipment Committee; past chair of the International Society for Respiratory Protection, Americas Section; secretariat chair of the ANSI Z88 for Respiratory Protection; and a member and secretary of the AIHA Respirator Committee. He is also a member of the AIHA Protective Clothing and Equipment Committees and the Emergency Preparedness and Response Task Force. Dr. Johnson retired from LLNL on July 1, 2006, and is now a part-time consultant.

JIMMY PERKINS, Ph.D., C.I.H., is professor of environmental and occupational health at the University of Texas School of Public Health. He received his B.A. at the University of Texas at Austin and his Ph.D. and M.S. in environmental health science at the University of Texas-Houston. Dr. Perkins served as a professor at the University of Alabama at Birmingham School of Public Health and has also worked in the petroleum industry and for the National Institute for Occupational Safety and Health (NIOSH). Dr. Perkins' research has focused on the permeation of chemicals through protective clothing and all aspects of dermal exposure risk management, including skin permeation models and mechanisms and the statistical aspects of chemical exposure assessment. Dr. Perkins is a certified industrial hygienist. He serves as a member of the IOM standing Committee on Personal Protective Equipment in the Workplace.

DAVID PREZANT, M.D., is the chief medical officer (Office of Medical Affairs) and senior pulmonary consultant to the New York City Fire Department (FDNY) and is professor of medicine at Albert Einstein College of Medicine and research director for the Pulmonary Division. He received his bachelor of science from Columbia College in 1977 and his doctor of medicine from Albert Einstein College of Medicine in 1981. Dr. Prezant is board-certified in internal medicine, pulmonary medicine, and critical care medicine. He is a member of the John P. Redmond IAFF Medical Advisory Board and represents FDNY as a member of the technical committee for the Fire Service Joint Labor Management Wellness-Fitness Initiative. Dr. Prezant is co-director of the NIOSH-funded FDNY World Trade Center Monitoring and Treatment Programs and is principal investigator for their Data Coordinating Center.

KNUT RINGEN, Dr.P.H., is a private consultant in disease management; environment, safety, and health risk management; workers' compensation; and group health insurance. Dr. Ringen specializes in the development of research and service programs, with an emphasis on workers and other special populations, and has been instrumental in developing many health programs that have achieved national significance. He has served as the director of the Center to Protect Workers' Rights and executive director of the Laborers' National Health and Safety Fund. Among many honors, he has been elected to the European Academy of Sciences and the Collegium Ramazzini. He received his doctor of public health degree from Johns Hopkins University for his research on the development of health policy, a master's degree in hospital administration from the Medical College of Virginia, and a master of public health degree from Johns Hopkins University. Dr. Ringen served as a member of the IOM Committee on the Assessment of the NIOSH Head-and-Face Anthropometric Survey of U.S. Respirator Users.

EMANUEL P. RIVERS, M.D., M.P.H., is vice chairman and director of research for the department of emergency medicine and senior staff attending physician in the Surgical Critical Care Unit and the Emergency Department at Henry Ford Hospital in Detroit, Michigan. Dr. Rivers received his master of public health and doctorate of medicine degrees from the University of Michigan in Ann Arbor. He completed a residency in emergency and internal medicine at Henry Ford Hospital, followed by a fellowship in cardiac critical care medicine at the University of Pittsburgh. He is board-certified in critical care medicine, emergency medicine, and internal medicine. Dr. Rivers is a fellow and recipient of a national research award from the American College of Physicians, Society of Academic Emergency Medicine, and the American College of Chest Physicians. His research interests focus on early detection and treatment of shock, particularly sepsis. Dr. Rivers was elected a member of the Institute of Medicine in 2005.

JOSEPH J. SCHWERHA, M.D., M.P.H., is professor and director of the Occupational and Environmental Medicine Residency Program at the University of Pittsburgh Graduate School of Public Health. He received his bachelor's degree in chemistry from the University of Pittsburgh; master's degree in public health, specializing in environmental health and industrial hygiene, from the University of Michigan; and medical degree from West Virginia University. He is board-certified in occupational medicine by the American Board of Preventive Medicine. Dr. Schwerha was general manager of health services and medical director at U.S. Steel for 30 years. He was awarded the 2005 William S. Knudsen Award by the American College of Occupational and Environmental Medicine, an international medical society of more than 6,000 physicians and health professionals. Dr. Schwerha is a member of the IOM standing Committee on Personal Protective Equipment in the Workplace and serves on the Committee to Review the NIOSH Traumatic Injury Program.

ANUGRAH SHAW, Ph.D., a textile technologist, is a professor at the University of Maryland Eastern Shore (UMES) and has conducted research on protective clothing for pesticide applicators for more than two decades. Her research includes work related to standardization of test methods, development of performance specifications, and studies related to the development and evaluation of personal protective equipment for hot climates. Dr. Shaw was responsible for the creation of an extensive database that includes data for more than 130 fabrics that were evaluated at UMES. This database has been used to develop an online system for work and protective clothing. Dr. Shaw serves as the technical contact for ASTM and ISO standards and performance specifications for protective clothing for pesticide applicators, and as an ISO delegate for a subcommittee on protective clothing. She has presented at numerous national and international conferences, published in several refereed journals, and written a book chapter on the selection of personal protective equipment. She received her Ph.D. in textile technology from Texas Woman's University.

TONYA L. SMITH-JACKSON, Ph.D., is director of the Assessment and Cognitive Ergonomics Laboratory, associate professor of human factors engineering in the Grado Department of Industrial and Systems Engineering, and adjunct associate professor of psychology in the department of psychology at Virginia Tech. She received a Ph.D. degree in psychology-ergonomics from North Carolina State University in 1998. She is also director of the Human Factors Engineering and Ergonomics Center and associate director of the Center for Innovation in Construction Safety and Health at Virginia Tech. Her research interests range from safety information presentation and comprehension in occupational and recreational settings to cognitive ergonomics. She is on the editorial board of *Ergonomics in Design* and the *Journal of Experimental Psychology: Applied*. Dr. Smith-Jackson is president of the Safety Technical Group of the Human Factors and Ergonomics Society and is a past member of the ANSI Z535 Committee.

FRAMEWORK COMMITTEE LIAISON

SUSAN E. COZZENS, Ph.D., is a professor of public policy at the Georgia Institute of Technology and director of its Technology Policy and Assessment Center. She earned her Ph.D. in sociology from Columbia University. She is currently working on research in the fields of science, technology, and inequalities; she continues to work internationally on developing methods for research assessment, as well as science and technology indicators. Prior to joining the faculty at the Georgia Institute of Technology, she was director of the NSF Office of Policy Support. Dr. Cozzens has served as a consultant to numerous organizations, including the Office of Science and Technology Policy, National Science Foundation, Office of Technology Assessment, General Accounting Office, National Cancer Institute, National Institute on Aging, and National Institutes of Health (NIH). She has served on several NRC and IOM committees, including Evaluation of the Sea Grant Program Review Process, Assessment of Centers of Excellence Programs at NIH, and Research Standards and Practices to Prevent the Destructive Application of Biotechnology, and is currently a member of the Committee to Review the NIOSH Hearing Loss Research Program. Dr. Cozzens is the past editor of *Science, Technology, & Human Values* and the *Journal of the Society for Social Studies of Science*. She currently is the coeditor of *Research Evaluation*.

BOARD ON HEALTH SCIENCES POLICY LIAISON

MARTHA N. HILL, Ph.D., is dean and professor at the Johns Hopkins University School of Nursing. She holds joint appointments in the Bloomberg School of Public Health and the School of Medicine. Dr. Hill, the 1997-1998 president of the American Heart Association, is a fellow in the American Academy of Nursing and a member of the Institute of Medicine of the National Academy of Sciences. She serves on the IOM Board on Health Sciences Policy and was the co-vice chair of the IOM report *Unequal Treatment: Confronting Ethnic and Racial Disparities in Health Care*. Dr. Hill received her bachelor of science degree in nursing from Johns Hopkins University, her master's degree from the University of Pennsylvania, and her doctoral degree in behavioral sciences from the Johns Hopkins University School of Public Health. Dr. Hill is internationally known for her work and research in preventing and treating hypertension and its complications among underserved blacks, particularly among young, urban black men. She is an active investigator and consultant on several NIH-funded clinical trials. She has published extensively and serves on numerous review panels, editorial boards, and advisory committees including the Board of Directors of Research!America. Dr. Hill has also consulted on hypertension and other cardiovascular-related issues in countries outside the United States, including South Africa, Scotland, Israel, and Australia.